The Complete

Sports
Nutrition

Second edition

Anita Bean

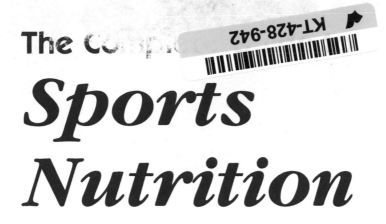

A & C Black · London

Contents

Also published by A & C Black:

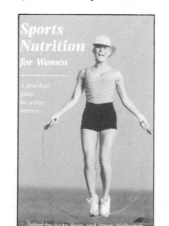

Sports Nutrition for Women

A practical guide for active women

Edited by Anita Bean and Peggy Wellington

Introduction

No matter what sport or exercise you do, you can improve your standard and get more out of your training by changing your diet. Good nutrition is vital for all sportspeople and fitness participants, whether you are an élite athlete, or simply keen to keep fit and healthy. What is eaten on a daily basis affects your energy levels, performance and overall health.

A deficiency in any particular nutrient or group of nutrients can hamper progress, while an optimal nutritional intake can be a distinct advantage. But what is an 'optimal' intake for sport? And how can it be achieved without spending a fortune? The aim of this book is to provide the answers to such questions, acting as a guide to the fascinating subject of sports nutrition by translating science into practical advice. It deals with key topics, such as energy and fatigue; 'carbing up'; losing and gaining weight; fluid intake; and what to eat for competition.

Controversial issues, such as protein requirements and the role of vitamins and minerals in exercise, are also covered. An in-depth look at sports supplements, pills, powders and drinks will help you to decide whether or not they live up to their claims. The relationship between body fat and sports performance is discussed along with the growing trend of eating disorders among athletes. There are plenty of strategies for weight loss, making weight for competition, and bulking up.

Vegetarian diets, calcium and bone health in female athletes, and snack-eating are also included. If you have to travel frequently or enjoy eating out in restaurants, eat on the run or dine late at night, this book shows how a nutritious diet can be maintained at home or away.

To anyone who is leading a busy life and following a hectic training schedule, eating a healthy diet must sound almost imposs-ible. Yet this is not so. By using this book you will be able to overcome any problems and enjoy good nutrition, even when you are busy. Good nutrition need not cost a fortune; there are lots of menu ideas and recipes in this book to help you eat well on a budget. Snack ideas and nutritious, easy-to-make recipes show that eating for sport can be fun, as well as healthy.

Good eating, and good training!

ANITA BEAN

Energise!
Fuels for exercise

When you exercise, your body must start producing energy very much faster than it does when it is at rest. The muscles start to contract more strenuously, the heart beats faster, pumping blood around the body more rapidly, and the lungs work harder. All these processes require extra energy. Where does it come from, and how can you make sure you have enough to last through a training session?

Before we can fully answer such questions, it is important to understand how the body produces energy, and what happens to it. This chapter looks at what takes place in the body when you exercise, where extra energy comes from, and how the fuel mixture used differs according to the type of exercise. It explains why fatigue occurs, how it can be delayed, and how you can get more out of training by changing your diet.

What is energy?

Although we cannot actually see energy, we can see and feel its effects in terms of heat and physical work. But what exactly is it?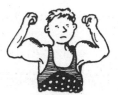

Energy is produced by the splitting of a chemical bond in a substance called *ATP* (adenosine triphosphate). This is often referred to as the body's 'energy currency'. It is produced in every cell of the body from the breakdown of carbohydrates, fats and proteins. These three fuels are transported and transformed by various biochemical processes into the same end product – ATP.

What is ATP?

ATP is a small molecule consisting of an adenosine 'backbone' with three phosphate groups attached.

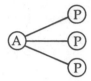

ADENOSINE TRIPHOSPHATE (ATP)

Energy is released when one of the phosphate groups splits off. When ATP loses one of its phosphate groups it becomes adenosine diphosphate, or *ADP*. Some energy is used to carry out work (such as muscle contractions), but most (around three-quarters) is given off as heat. This is why you feel warmer when you exercise. Once this has happened, ADP is converted back into ATP. A continual cycle takes place, in which ATP forms ADP and then becomes ATP again.

The inter-conversion of adenosine triphosphate and adenosine diphosphate

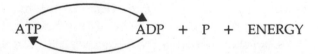

The body stores only very small amounts of ATP at any one time. There is just enough to keep up basic energy requirements while you are at rest — sufficient to keep the body ticking over. When you start exercising, energy demand suddenly increases, and the supply of ATP is used up within a few seconds. As more ATP must be produced to continue exercising, more fuel must be broken down.

Where does energy come from?

There are four components in food and drink that are capable of producing energy:

- carbohydrate
- fat
- protein
- alcohol

When you eat a meal or have a drink, these components are broken down in the digestive system into their various constituents or building blocks. Then they are absorbed into the bloodstream. Carbohydrates are broken down into small, single sugar units: glucose (the most common unit), fructose and galactose. Fats are broken down into fatty acids, and proteins into amino acids. Alcohol is mostly absorbed directly into the blood.

The ultimate fate of all of these components is energy production, although carbohydrates, proteins and fats also have other important functions.

Carbohydrates and alcohol are used mainly for energy in the short term, while fats are used as a long term energy store. Proteins can be used to produce energy either in 'emergencies' (for instance, when carbohydrates are in short supply) or when they have reached the end of their useful life. Sooner or later, all food and drink components are broken down to release energy.

How is energy measured?

Energy is ultimately given off from the body as heat. It is measured in units of heat, called joules. In scientific terms, 1 joule (J) is the energy used to move a weight of 1 kilogram (kg) over 1 metre (m) by a force of 1 newton (N). However, imperial units of energy, calories, are still used more commonly than joules. One calorie (cal) is defined as the amount of heat required to increase the temperature of 1 gram (g) of water by 1 degree centigrade (°C).

As the calorie and the joule represent very small amounts of energy, kilocalories (kcal or Cal) and kilojoules (kJ) are more often used. As their names suggest, a kilocalorie is 1,000 calories and a kilojoule 1,000 joules. You have probably seen these units on food labels. When we mention calories in the everyday sense, we are really talking about Calories with a capital C, or kilocalories (kcal or Cal).

To convert kilocalories into kilojoules, simply multiply by 4.2. For example:

1 kcal = 4.2 kJ
10 kcal = 42 kJ

To convert kilojoules into kilocalories, divide by 4.2. For example, if 100 g of food provides 400 kJ, and you wish to know how many kilocalories that is, divide 400 by 4.2 to find the equivalent number of kilocalories:

400 kJ ÷ 4.2 = 95 kcal

Why do different foods provide different amounts of energy?

Foods are made of different amounts of carbohydrates, fats, proteins and alcohol. Each of these nutrients provides a certain quantity of energy when it is broken down in the body. For instance, 1 g of carbohydrate or protein releases about 4 kcal of energy, while 1 g of fat releases 9 kcal, and 1 g of alcohol releases 7 kcal.

The energy value of different food components

1 g provides:

- ◆ carbohydrate   16 kJ (4 kcal)
- ◆ fat   37 kJ (9 kcal)
- ◆ protein   17 kJ (4 kcal)
- ◆ alcohol   23 kJ (7 kcal).

Fat is the most concentrated form of energy, providing the body with more than twice as much energy as carbohydrate or protein, and also more than alcohol. However, it is not necessarily the 'best' form of energy for exercise.

All foods contain a mixture of nutrients, and the energy value of a particular food depends on the amount of carbohydrate, fat and protein it contains. For example, one slice of wholemeal bread provides roughly the same amount of energy as one pat (7 g) of butter. However, their composition is very different. In bread, most energy (75%) comes from carbohydrate, while in butter, virtually all (99.7%) comes from fat.

How does my body store carbohydrate?

Carbohydrate is stored as *glycogen* in the muscles and liver, along .h about three times its own weight of water. Altogether there is

Table 1: *The measurement of energy*

To find the percentage of energy from carbohydrate:

$$\frac{\text{g carbohydrate} \times 4}{\text{Total calories}} \times 100\% \quad = \% \text{ energy from carbohydrate}$$

To find the percentage of energy from fat:

$$\frac{\text{g fat} \times 9}{\text{Total calories}} \times 100\% \quad = \% \text{ energy from fat}$$

To find the percentage of energy from protein:

$$\frac{\text{g protein} \times 4}{\text{Total calories}} \times 100\% \quad = \% \text{ energy from protein}$$

To find the percentage of energy from alcohol:

$$\frac{\text{g alcohol} \times 7}{\text{Total calories}} \times 100\% \quad = \% \text{ energy from alcohol}$$

---

about three times more glycogen stored in the muscles than in the liver. Glycogen is a large molecule, similar to starch, made up of many glucose units joined together. However, the body can store only a relatively small amount of glycogen – there is no endless supply! Like the petrol tank in a car, the body can only hold a certain amount.

The total store of glycogen in the average body amounts to about 1600–2000 kcal – enough to last one day if you were to eat nothing. This is why a low carbohydrate diet tends to make people lose quite a lot of weight in the first few days. The weight loss is almost entirely due to loss of glycogen and water.

Table 2: *Fuel reserves in a person weighing 70 kg* [1]

Fuel stores	Potential energy available (kcal)		
	Glycogen	**Fats**	**Proteins**
Liver	400	450	400
Adipose tissue (fat)	0	135,000	0
Muscle	1,200	350	24,000

1 Cahill, GF (1976). *Starvation in man.* J Clin Endocrinol Metab 5, 397–415.

Small amounts of glucose are present in the blood (approximately 15 g, which is equivalent to 60 kcal) and in the brain (about 2 g or 8 kcal) and their concentrations are kept within a very narrow range, both at rest and during exercise. This allows normal body functions to continue.

How does my body store fat?

Fat is stored as *adipose* (fat) tissue in almost every region of the body. A small amount of fat is stored in muscles – this is called intramuscular fat – but the majority is stored around the organs and beneath the skin. The amount stored in different parts of the body depends on genetic make-up and individual hormone balance. Interestingly, people who store fat mostly around their abdomen (the classic pot belly shape) have a higher risk of heart disease than those who store fat mostly around their hips and thighs (the classic pear shape).

Unfortunately, there is little you can do to change the way that your body distributes fat. But you can definitely change the *amount* of fat that is stored, as you will see in Chapter 7.

You will probably find that your basic shape is similar to that of one or both of your parents. Males usually take after their father, and females after their mother. Female hormones tend to favour fat storage around the hips and thighs, while male hormones encourage fat storage around the middle. This is why, in general, women are 'pear shaped' and men are 'apple shaped'.

How does my body store protein?

Protein is not stored in the same way as carbohydrate and fat. It forms muscle and organ tissue, so it is mainly used as a building material rather than an energy store. However, proteins *can* be broken down to release energy if need be, so muscles and organs represent a large source of *potential* energy.

Which fuels are most important for exercise?

Carbohydrates, fats and proteins are all capable of providing energy for exercise; they can all be transported to, and broken down in, muscle cells. Alcohol, however, cannot be used directly by muscles for energy during exercise, no matter how strenuously they may be working. Only the liver has the specific enzymes needed to break down alcohol. You cannot break down alcohol faster by exercising harder either – the liver carries out its job at a fixed speed. Do not think you can work off a few drinks by going for a jog, or by drinking a cup of black coffee!

Proteins do not make a substantial contribution to the fuel mixture. It is only during very prolonged or very intense bouts of exercise that proteins play a more important role in giving the body energy.

The production of ATP during most forms of exercise comes mainly from broken down carbohydrates and fats.

When is protein used for energy?

Protein is not usually a major source of energy, but it may play a more important role during the latter stages of very strenuous or prolonged exercise as glycogen stores become depleted. For example, during the last stages of a marathon or a long distance cycle race, when glycogen stores are exhausted, the proteins in muscles (and organs) may make up around 10% of the body's fuel mixture.

During a period of semi starvation, or if a person follows a low carbohydrate diet, glycogen would be in short supply, so more proteins would be broken down to provide the body with fuel. Up to half of the weight lost by someone following a low calorie or low carbohydrate diet comes from protein (muscle) loss. Some people think that if they deplete their glycogen stores by following a low carbohydrate diet, they will force their body to break down more fat and lose weight. This is not the case: you risk losing muscle as well as fat, and there are many other disadvantages, too. These are discussed in Chapter 8.

How does my body decide which fuel to use?

The amount of each fuel that your muscles use during exercise depends on the following:

◆ type, duration and intensity of exercise
◆ fitness level and training programme
◆ diet and nutritional status.

The fuel mixture used for a short sprint differs from that used for a long, slow jog. In other words, a different 'blend' of carbohydrate/ fat/protein is used when you sprint than when you jog. The fuel blend also changes as the exercise continues: the combination used at the start will be different from that used at the end. Also, a fit, highly trained athlete would have a different fuel blend from a beginner.

How does the intensity of my training affect my fuel mixture?

Generally speaking, as you exercise harder, you use a greater proportion of carbohydrate and a smaller proportion of fat.

Figure 1: *Fuel mixture and exercise intensity*

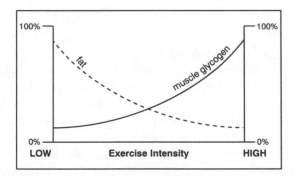

During light or low intensity aerobic exercise (such as walking or jogging), both carbohydrate and fat are used. As, for example, you slow down from a fast jog to a slow jog, you will use a greater percentage of fat, a smaller percentage of carbohydrate, and fewer calories.

As you increase your pace, i.e. as the intensity of the exercise increases, your body will gradually use a smaller percentage of fat, a greater percentage of carbohydrate for ATP production, and more calories.

During moderate or high intensity aerobic exercise, such as fast running, only a small proportion of the body's fuel mixture comes from fat. Most comes from carbohydrates.

During extremely high intensity anaerobic exercise, such as sprinting, carbohydrates will be a major source of fuel, and no energy will come from fat.

Is low intensity exercise better for burning fat?

Not necessarily! Although fat provides a greater percentage of energy during low intensity exercise, you still have to take account of the total calories burned. For example, walking for 60 minutes burns 270 kcal, of which 60% (160 kcal) comes from fat. However, jogging for 60 minutes burns 680 kcal, of which 40% (270 kcal) comes from fat. Thus the higher intensity exercise results in a greater fat loss over the same period of time.

As shown in Table 3, a shorter period (e.g. 40 min) of high intensity exercise burns about the same amount of fat as a longer period (e.g. 60 min) of low intensity exercise. So, if time is a premium, shorter periods of high intensity exercise will give you the same results in terms of fat loss as longer periods of low intensity exercise.

On the other hand, low intensity exercise is often more suitable for beginners as they may not be fit enough to embark on a high intensity programme. Also, low intensity exercise is more accessible and enjoyable for many people and, therefore, they are more likely to continue the exercise programme.

In summary, if fat loss is your main goal, choose high intensity aerobic exercise if you are sufficiently fit and enjoy doing it or if you have relatively little time to work out. Choose longer periods of low intensity exercise if you are less fit and prefer it to high intensity exercise.

Table 3: *Calorie and fat burning during low and high intensity exercise*

Exercise	Distance (miles)	Speed (mph)	Duration (min)	Total calories* (kcal)	Calories from fat (%)	(kcal)
Walking	4	4	60	270	60	160
Jogging	4	6	40	450	40	180
Jogging	6	6	60	680	40	270

* Based on ACSM Guidelines for Exercise Testing & Prescription (1991)

How does the duration of exercise affect my fuel mixture?

As you continue to exercise aerobically, you use more and more fat and less and less carbohydrate. In fact, the body will make every effort to conserve its carbohydrate (glycogen) stores.

Figure 2: *Fuel mixture and exercise duration*

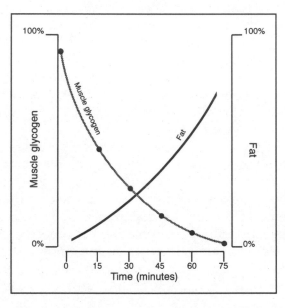

Fat is never burned completely on its own. Certain substances that are produced by the breaking down of carbohydrates are essential if fat is also to be broken down. There must always be at least a small amount of carbohydrate present to help the body burn fat. Fat burns in the fire of carbohydrate.

Glycogen in the muscles is unable to provide energy indefinitely. For example, you have enough glycogen to last just 90–180 minutes of endurance exercise at 60–80% of your maximal aerobic capacity (e.g. cycling); or 30–45 minutes of high intensity/ anaerobic activities (e.g. weight training); or 45–90 minutes of endurance/anaerobic activity (e.g. football). During the later stages of endurance events (such as long distance running or cycling), the glycogen stores in muscles are very depleted. At this stage, the glycogen stores in the liver become more important. Muscle proteins start to break down into amino acids to help meet energy demands and, after three or four hours of exercise (such as during the last stages of a marathon), 75–90% of the carbohydrate used by the muscles may be coming from glucose released by the liver. Some of this glucose comes from glycogen, but some also comes from other substances, such as amino acids and lactic acid. These are converted into carbohydrate in the liver.

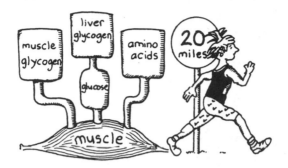

All these energy producing systems keep glucose levels steady in the blood. In fact, the level is kept within a surprisingly narrow range, despite continual energy demands. However, after very long periods of exercise of three hours or more (when liver and muscle glycogen stores become very depleted), glucose levels in the blood can drop below the normal range. This condition is known as hypoglycaemia. It causes fatigue, nausea and dizziness.

How does my fitness level affect the fuel mixture?

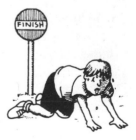

As a result of aerobic training, muscles become better at using fat and sparing glycogen. This means that the body is able to exercise for longer before glycogen stores run down and fatigue sets in.

The fitter you are, the lower the proportion of glycogen and the higher the proportion of fat your muscles will use at any given exercise intensity. If a trained athlete and a beginner exercised at the same intensity, the trained athlete would use less glycogen and more fat at any given time and therefore experience fatigue later than the beginner. This is one of the natural adaptations to aerobic training – your body becomes more efficient in breaking down fats, transporting and oxidising the fatty acids and develops greater numbers of fat-oxidising enzymes (*see* fig. 3).

Figure 3: *Trained people use less glycogen and more fat*

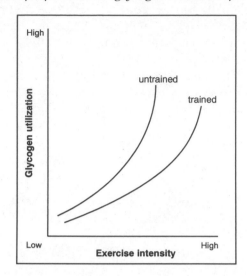

What is the difference between anaerobic and aerobic exercise?

Exercise is often broadly classified as either aerobic or anaerobic. Aerobic literally means 'with oxygen'; anaerobic 'without oxygen'.

In practice, most activities are unlikely to be purely aerobic or anaerobic, although usually one system is dominant. Examples of anaerobic activities include sprinting, throwing, jumping, kicking and weight training. In other words, these are activities of high intensity and short duration. The body must produce energy very rapidly without the help of oxygen. Since oxygen is not present, these forms of activity can only be kept up for a very brief period.

Examples of aerobic activities include walking, jogging, long distance cycling, swimming and exercise to music – even sitting and standing! These are of low intensity and longer duration. Energy is produced in the presence of oxygen, and the activity can therefore be kept up for much longer than in an anaerobic situation.

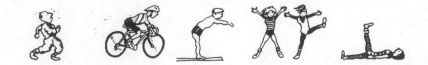

What happens in my body during anaerobic activity?

During anaerobic activity, carbohydrate must be converted into energy very quickly in order to meet sudden and massive energy demands. Such demands occur when you lift, jump, kick, hit, sprint or throw – movements included in many sports.

In order to meet these sudden, huge demands, glucose bypasses the energy producing pathways that would normally use oxygen, and follows a different route that does not use oxygen. This saves a good deal of time.

Instead of making the usual 38 molecules of ATP per glucose molecule, the body can make only two ATP molecules using its anaerobic response, because glucose is only *partially* broken down in these conditions. It is converted into lactic acid, instead of carbon dioxide and water (*see* fig. 4).

In order to generate a sufficiently large amount of ATP, a lot of glucose must be broken down. The body's glycogen stores dwindle quite quickly, proving that the benefits of a fast delivery service come at a price.

Figure 4: *Anaerobic energy system*

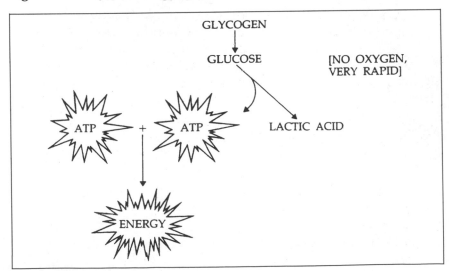

Unfortunately, producing ATP as rapidly as this cannot be kept up for very long – 90 seconds at most. This is due to a build-up of lactic acid, a by-product of this rapid means of glucose breakdown. Lactic acid prevents the production of further energy by creating an acidic environment in the body that eventually hinders the contractions of the muscles. For this reason no one can keep running or cycling at an all-out pace for very long.

What happens to my body during aerobic activity?

During aerobic exercise ATP is produced along the more usual route, using oxygen, and glucose is *completely* broken down into carbon dioxide, water and energy (*see* fig. 5). Down the anaerobic route, glucose is only *partially* broken down, and no carbon dioxide or water is produced.

In aerobic exercise, the demand for energy is slower and smaller than in an anaerobic activity, so there is more time to transport sufficient oxygen from the lungs to the muscles and for glucose to generate ATP with the help of the oxygen. Under these circumstances, one molecule of glucose can create up to 38 molecules of ATP. Thus, aerobic energy production is about 20 times more efficient than anaerobic energy production.

Anaerobic exercise uses only glycogen, whereas aerobic exercise uses both glycogen and fat, so can be kept up for longer though the disadvantage is that it produces energy more slowly.

Fats can also be used to produce energy in the aerobic system. One fatty acid can produce between 80 and 200 ATP molecules, depending on its type. Fats are therefore an even more efficient energy source than carbohydrates. However, they can only be broken down into ATP under aerobic conditions when energy demands are relatively low, and so energy production is slower.

Figure 5: *Aerobic energy system*

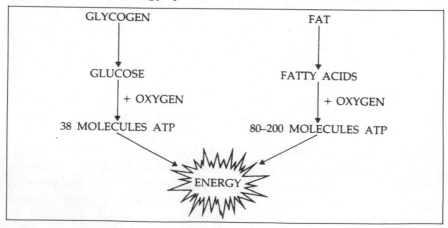

What happens to lactic acid?

Lactic acid produced by muscles under anaerobic conditions does not stay around for long – otherwise you would not be able to move again! When the exercise intensity is reduced (e.g. slowing from a fast run to a slow jog), lactic acid can be removed from muscle cells. This can only happen if enough oxygen is present.

Lactic acid may be converted into another substance, called pyruvic acid, which can then change into ATP when there is enough oxygen around (i.e. it regenerates energy). This can happen in the same muscle cell or in neighbouring cells within the same muscle.

Alternatively, lactic acid may be carried away from the muscle in the bloodstream to the liver, where it can be converted back into glucose, released into the bloodstream and then taken back to the same muscle. Here it can be used either to produce more energy or, if the muscle is at rest, to make glycogen again.

Is lactic acid always produced?

Lactic acid is produced during most types of exercise, not just anaerobic. An exception is the sort of explosive activity resulting from a single lift during weight training or a 20-metre dash during a football match. In these cases, existing supplies of ATP and phosphocreatine, or PC, (*see* page 20) are sufficient for the energy demand. No glycogen is needed and no lactic acid produced.

During low intensity aerobic exercise, such as an easy jog or brisk walk, lactic acid is produced slowly from glycogen/glucose and is removed before it can build up. In other words, clearance keeps pace with production and does not interfere with the creation of energy. As the intensity of an exercise increases (for example, from a brisk walk to a jog and then a sprint), more and more lactic acid is produced.

When the body can no longer remove lactic acid as fast as it is produced (for instance during very strenuous exercise), the acid starts to build up, eventually preventing energy production and muscle movement. The exercise has to stop or slow down.

If the intensity of an exercise is reduced, by slowing down or resting, more oxygen is available to the muscle. This means that the lactic acid can be removed and exercise can continue. Slowing down like this is sometimes called 'repaying the oxygen debt'.

More about the anaerobic energy system

The anaerobic energy system can be divided into two parts: the **phosphocreatine system** (PC); and the **lactic acid system** (LA). Both occur during anaerobic conditions (without oxygen), and both are used to create ATP (energy) very quickly indeed.

1 The PC system

This system of regenerating ATP is used for fast, sudden bursts of activity lasting just a few seconds; for example, in a single throw, jump or lift, or in a 20-metre sprint. The PC system can be thought of as a back-up to ATP, as it helps to regenerate ATP from ADP. It possesses a high energy phosphate bond which can break off and transfer to a molecule of ADP, making a new ATP molecule very quickly. The supply of PC is limited and can last only for a few seconds, providing about 3 or 4 kcal. After this, it must be regenerated from other fuels, such as glycogen or fats. When this happens, other systems take over.

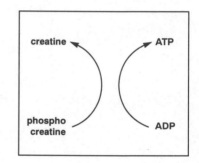

2 The LA system

The LA system is used almost exclusively during events such as the 400 and 800 metres, during weight training (for a set of 8–15 repetitions taken to failure), or for any other burst of all-out activity lasting about 90 seconds. The fuel is glycogen or glucose, which rapidly (but incompletely) breaks down without oxygen to form lactic acid, and produces two molecules of ATP for every glucose molecule. The gradual build-up of lactic acid in the body eventually prevents muscle contractions.

It is important to note that neither of these anaerobic systems are confined to high intensity activities. They are used, to a lesser extent, in most other forms of exercise; in aerobic sports, such as long distance running, and in intermittent sports, such as football.

Table 4: Energy systems

| | ANAEROBIC (without oxygen) | | AEROBIC (with oxygen) |
	PC system	LA system	
Intensity	very high, explosive 95–100% max effort	high 60–95% max effort	low up to 60% max effort
Duration	up to 10 sec	up to 30 sec (95% max effort) up to 30 min (60% max effort)	no limit
Fuel	phospho-creatine (PC)	muscle glycogen +blood glucose	carbohydrate +fat +protein
Waste product	none	lactic acid	$CO_2 + H_2O$
Recovery time	very quick (30 sec–2 min)	20 min–2 hours	time to replace fuel stores

Is my sport aerobic or anaerobic?

No sport can be strictly classified as either aerobic or anaerobic, although as a general rule the faster you are moving, the more likely you are to be burning carbohydrate and less likely to be burning fat. Sports that involve short, sharp bursts of activity, such as throwing and sprinting, are predominantly anaerobic.

In practice, though, most sports are a mixture of both aerobic and anaerobic activity. For example, in football, hockey and rugby there are short bursts of very strenuous activity (sprints, kicks, throws, etc.) interspersed with longer periods of less strenuous activity (such as jogging and walking).

Endurance sports, such as long distance running, swimming and cycling, are predominantly aerobic. They involve relatively slow, rhythmical movements which can be sustained for long periods. The supply of oxygen to muscles is more in keeping with energy demands, and the body can burn a mixture of both fat and carbohydrate.

Figure 6: *Percentage contribution of energy systems during exercise of different durations*

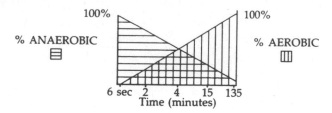

Table 5: *Aerobic and anaerobic exercise*

	ANAEROBIC	**AEROBIC**
Examples of activity	Weight lifting Sprinting Gymnastics Squash Badminton Judo/karate Discus/shot put High/long jump	Jogging Distance running Distance cycling Distance swimming Exercise to music Distance rowing Brisk walking Skiing
Fuel used	Mostly carbohydrate	Fat + carbohydrate
Rate of energy production	Rapid	Slow
Duration	0–90 sec	Up to several hours

What happens in my body when I start exercising?

When you begin to exercise, energy is produced without oxygen for at least the first few seconds, before your breathing rate and heart can catch up with energy demands. Therefore, a build-up of lactic acid takes place. As the heart and lungs work harder, getting more oxygen into your body, carbohydrates and fats can be broken down aerobically. If you are exercising fairly gently (i.e. your oxygen supply keeps up with your energy demands), any lactic acid that accumulated earlier can be removed easily since there is now enough oxygen around.

If you continue to exercise aerobically, more oxygen is delivered around the body and more fats start to be broken down into fatty acids. They are taken to muscle cells via the bloodstream and then broken down with oxygen to produce energy.

In effect, the anaerobic system 'buys time' in the first few minutes of an exercise, before the body's slower aerobic system can start to function.

For the first 5–15 minutes of exercise (depending on your aerobic fitness level) the main fuel is carbohydrate (glycogen). As time goes on, however, more oxygen is delivered to the muscles, and you will use proportionally less carbohydrate and more fat.

On the other hand, if you begin exercising very strenuously (e.g. by running fast), lactic acid quickly builds up in the muscles. The delivery of oxygen cannot keep pace with the huge energy demand, so lactic acid continues to accumulate and very soon you will feel fatigue. You must then either slow down and run more slowly, or stop. Nobody can maintain a fast run for very long.

If you start a distance race or training run too fast, you will suffer from fatigue early on and be forced to reduce your pace considerably. A head start will not necessarily give any benefit at all. Warm up *before* the start of a race (by walking, slow jogging, or performing gentle mobility exercises), so that the heart and lungs can start to work a little harder, and oxygen delivery to the muscles can increase. Start the race at a moderate pace, gradually building up to an optimal speed. This will prevent a large 'oxygen debt' and avoid an early depletion of glycogen. In this way, your optimal pace can be sustained for longer.

The anaerobic system can also 'cut in' to help energy production, for instance when the demand for energy temporarily exceeds the body's oxygen supply. If you run uphill at the same pace as on the flat, your energy demand increases. The body will generate extra energy by breaking down glycogen/glucose anaerobically. However, this can only be kept up for a short period of time, because there will be a gradual build-up of lactic acid. The lactic acid can be removed aerobically afterwards, by running back down the hill, for example.

The same principle applies during fast bursts of activity in interval training, when energy is produced anaerobically. Lactic acid accumulates and is then removed during the rest interval.

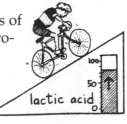

lactic acid

How much fat can I expect to burn?

The speed at which your body can produce energy from fats, and the amount it can produce, depends on a number of things.

1 How fast your body can break down fats in adipose tissue into their component fatty acids. This requires oxygen, so you must be exercising aerobically.
2 How fast your body can deliver these fatty acids into muscle cells elsewhere in your body.
3 How fast the fatty acids are transported from the main area of the muscle cell into the little 'power houses' within the muscle cells (the mitochondria).
4 How many mitochondria there are in the muscle cells.
5 The number of fat burning enzymes in your mitochondria.
6 The proportion of muscle fibre types in your body. Different types of fibre are better suited to producing ATP aerobically or anaerobically. This is largely genetic, although it can be partially influenced by training.

Each of these factors can be improved and made more efficient by regular aerobic training. Over a period of time, aerobic training will make it easier for the body to break down fat and use it as energy during aerobic exercise. In other words, regular aerobic training makes a person a more efficient 'fat burner'. The body can then break down fats into fatty acids more readily, deliver them to muscle cells faster (because the number of blood capillaries serving

Table 6: *Depletion of fuel reserves during different types of exercise*

Fuel	Maximal, short bursts	High intensity, intermittent	High intensity, < 40 min
PC	Great	Very great	Moderate
Muscle glycogen	Slight	Moderate	Moderate
Liver glycogen + blood glucose	Negligible	Slight	Slight
Fat	Negligible	Slight	Negligible

Fuel	High intensity, 40–150 min	High intensity, > 150 min	Low intensity
PC	Moderate	Moderate	Negligible
Muscle glycogen	Very great	Very great	Negligible
Liver glycogen + blood glucose	Moderate – great	Great – very great	Slight
Fat	Negligible	Slight	Slight

($<$ = less than, $>$ = more than)

the muscle increases), and also transport the fatty acids faster into the mitochondria. The number of mitochondria and fat burning enzymes within them also increases. This helps to make the fat preferring muscle fibres work more efficiently.

So, at any given exercise intensity (even at rest), the fitter you are, the more fat and the less glycogen your body will use. This is important because glycogen is in much shorter supply than fat. By using fat you can make your body's valuable glycogen stores last longer and thereby delay fatigue.

Regular aerobic exercise can therefore increase the body's efficiency in terms of energy production, and help to keep body fat levels within a healthy range. This is why fat endurance athletes are few and far between! In contrast, athletes involved in anaerobic sports, such as power lifting or shot putting, often have higher body fat levels due to a lack of aerobic training.

What is fatigue?

Fatigue during exercise can be experienced in many forms. In ball games, such as football, tennis and hockey, you may find it harder to sprint for the ball, despite being able to jog at the general playing pace. When you do get there, you may not be able to strike the ball as hard as before. In martial arts, you may notice that your reaction times are slower and your co-ordination and balance skills poorer. Concentration may falter in team sports, and in athletic events, technique or form may suffer in the latter stages. In aerobics classes, you may find it hard to maintain pace or technique.

You should now be able to recognise fatigue!

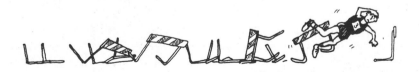

Why do I experience fatigue during exercise?

Fatigue may be due to a number of factors, depending largely on the type of exercise.

1 Aerobic exercise

Fatigue during moderate to high intensity aerobic exercise, such as running, cycling and swimming, occurs when muscle glycogen stores have run down. It is like running out of petrol in a car. At this point, it is not possible to maintain the same exercise intensity (e.g. a running pace). You will either have to reduce the exercise intensity (e.g. by running at a slower pace), or stop.

The fitter you are, the longer it takes for your glycogen stores to become depleted. An unfit person will run out of muscle glycogen ('petrol') faster than a fit person, and will therefore suffer fatigue sooner.

Figure 7: *The increase in perceived exertion as glycogen stores become depleted*

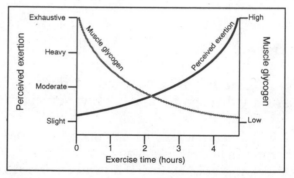

As we have already seen, fatigue after long periods (three hours or more) of low to moderate intensity exercise is due to depleted muscle *and* liver glycogen stores and low blood glucose levels. On the other hand, after very long periods of low intensity exercise (e.g. walking for several hours) fatigue is more likely to be related to a rise in a brain chemical called serotonin, which is responsible for sleepiness and mood. This type of fatigue is called *central fatigue*, i.e. related to the brain and central nervous system.

However, during higher intensity aerobic exercise, such as a 10 km race, fatigue is normally due both to depleted muscle glycogen stores and a build-up of lactic acid. Very little liver glycogen is used in these conditions, so fatigue is not due to low liver glycogen stores or low blood glucose levels. The amount of time that a person can spend exercising at this intensity is obviously limited – about 90 minutes is the most that well trained individuals can manage (equivalent to a half marathon). Less fit people are unable to exercise at this intensity for very long.

2 Anaerobic exercise

During explosive maximal activities, fatigue is usually due to PC depletion. During most anaerobic exercise, though, it is caused by a rapid build-up of lactic acid, causing you to feel pain or unable to move your muscles. However, if you reduce the intensity of the exercise or take a short rest, the lactic acid can be cleared and you can repeat the exercise bout. It is actually impossible to continue high intensity exercises indefinitely, since the acid environment that would be created in your muscles would eventually prove fatal! The feeling of pain when lactic acid is present is a kind of safety mechanism, preventing the body from self destruction.

As the body relies almost entirely on its muscle glycogen stores to provide energy, a further cause of fatigue is low stores of glycogen. By the end of a training session a person's muscle glycogen stores are considerably depleted.

No matter what type of exercise you do or how fit you are, your body will always use glycogen. The amount of glycogen that is in the muscles (and, in some cases, the liver) *before* exercise begins is of key importance. The size of your glycogen stores is therefore a limiting factor in exercise performance. The larger the pre-exercise glycogen stores, the longer you will be able to exercise before experiencing fatigue.

So, if you want to get the most out of training sessions and perform at your best in competitions, the message is: *always start exercise with 'full' glycogen stores.*

Finally, beware of dehydration, another major cause of fatigue, which is discussed further in Chapter 6.

How can I delay fatigue?

You can help to delay fatigue in the following ways.

1 Start exercising with full glycogen stores

Think of it like setting off on a car journey with a full tank of petrol. The more you have to start with, the longer you can keep going. If you set off on your journey with only half a tank of petrol, you will either have to stop halfway or slow down to a more economical speed to conserve what little petrol you have. Instead of driving to your destination at 70 mph, you may have to slow down to a more economical 56 mph.

In other words, if you start exercising with full glycogen stores, you will be able to run faster for longer or lift heavier weights for more repetitions and more sets. You will also find that fatigue is delayed.

2 Reduce the rate at which you use up muscle glycogen

The rate at which you use glycogen depends on a number of things: the type and intensity of the exercise you are doing; your fitness level; and the temperature of surroundings (if you are exercising in hot weather, you will tend to use more glycogen than in cold weather).

Try to pace yourself. Build up exercise intensity gradually, as this will help you to eke out your glucose supply over a longer period of time. If you start off too fast you will use up too much glycogen too soon and suffer fatigue earlier.

How does diet help to delay fatigue?

A diet that is rich in carbohydrates will ensure high glycogen stores. Remember that glycogen is made up of glucose that is derived from carbohydrates in your diet. If you eat a high carbohydrate diet, your muscle and liver glycogen stores are more likely to be 'full'. This will help you to continue exercising for longer and to perform at your best.

Relationship between muscle glycogen and exercise

The importance of carbohydrates in relation to exercise performance was first demonstrated in 1939 by two researchers, Christensen and Hansen. They found that a high carbohydrate diet significantly increased endurance. However, it was not until the 1960s that the relationship between muscle glycogen and exercise was fully investigated. Scandinavian research groups demonstrated that as exercise increases in intensity, the body requires more muscle glycogen, and that fatigue is related to depleted stores. They discovered that the capacity to perform aerobic exercise was related to the initial size of a person's muscle glycogen stores, and that a high carbohydrate diet can increase endurance.

Case Study

In a famous study by Bergstrom and his colleagues, groups of athletes were fed on a low carbohydrate diet (LC), on a high carbohydrate diet (HC), or on a normal mixed diet (M) [2]. Researchers measured the concentration of glycogen in their leg muscles and found that those eating the HC diet had twice as much glycogen as those eating the M diet, and seven times more than those on the LC diet! Afterwards the athletes exercised on a stationary bike, at an intensity equivalent to 75% of their maximal aerobic capacity, until they became exhausted. Those on the HC diet managed to cycle for 170 minutes, far longer than those on the M diet, who managed 115 minutes, and those on the LC diet, who cycled for 60 minutes. The experiment showed that there is a direct connection between glycogen levels before exercise and the performance of an exercise.

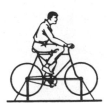

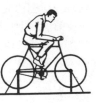

NORMAL MIXED DIET

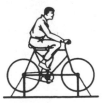
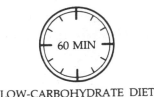
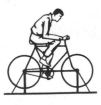

LOW-CARBOHYDRATE DIET

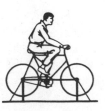
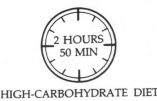
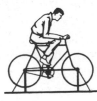

HIGH-CARBOHYDRATE DIET

2 Bergstrom, J *et al.* (1967). *Diet, muscle glycogen and physical performance.* Acta Physiol Scand *71*, 140–150.

SUMMARY OF KEY POINTS

- Energy for exercise is provided by three main fuels: carbohydrate, fat and protein, each yielding 4 kcal/g, 9 kcal/g and 4 kcal/g respectively.
- The amount and proportion of each fuel used depends on the type, duration and intensity of exercise; your fitness level; and your diet.
- For aerobic activities, all three fuels may be broken down (although protein makes a significantly smaller contribution than fat and glycogen). For anaerobic activities, only phosphocreatine (PC) and glycogen are broken down.
- The proportion of carbohydrate (glycogen) used increases with exercise intensity and decreases with exercise duration.
- The main cause of fatigue during aerobic exercise is usually glycogen depletion and/or dehydration. The main cause of fatigue during anaerobic exercise is initially PC depletion and/or lactic acid build up but, after several sets/bouts, fatigue is eventually also due to glycogen depletion.
- For almost all types of exercise, performance is limited by the amount of glycogen in the muscles. Low pre-exercise stores lead to early fatigue, reduced training intensity and reduced training gains.
- Ensuring full glycogen stores before each training session can help delay fatigue and improve performance. This can be achieved by a high carbohydrate diet.

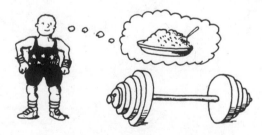

Carbo power

Carbohydrate and fat can both be used as fuels by exercising muscles. However, as we saw in the last chapter, requirements vary according to the type of exercise involved, the intensity and duration of a training session, and individual fitness levels.

One thing is clear, though: no matter what the type of exercise, you will always be using some glycogen. You cannot exercise without it. The amount of glycogen in your muscles will dictate how hard and how long you can exercise for. Low glycogen levels will lead to early fatigue. High glycogen levels, on the other hand, mean you can train harder and for longer.

Clearly, then, glycogen is the most important and most valuable fuel for any type of exercise. This chapter explains what happens if you fail to eat enough carbohydrate and glycogen levels become depleted. It shows how you can fuel up with glycogen between training sessions and make sure that you have the maximum energy available for each session. Different types of carbohydrate produce different responses in the body, so this chapter also gives advice on which carbohydrates to eat, how much and how often, as well as presenting the latest thinking on 'carb loading' before a competition.

Why should I refuel?

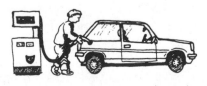

By the end of an exercise session your muscle glycogen stores will be lower than when you started.

Think of a long car journey: when you set out you have a full tank of petrol, and at the end it is nearly empty. To make another journey, you have to fill up with petrol and replace the fuel you have just used up. Obviously, if you do not do this you will not be able to make your next journey!

In the same way, you have to refuel your body's glycogen stores after training in order to replace the energy that you have just used up. If not, you will turn up at your next training session with low glycogen stores.

How will I feel with low glycogen stores?

Training with low glycogen stores means that you will experience fatigue more quickly and find it harder to continue exercising at the same intensity. Your workout becomes less intense, your technique will suffer and chances of injury increase. If this continues for consecutive workouts over a period of time, you will eventually develop symptoms of over training – reduced training stimulus and gains; chronic fatigue; and decreased immune system. It's like taking your car out on a second journey without putting enough petrol back in the tank – you will not be able to drive as far and may have to slow down to a more economical speed, ending up at your destination later than planned (if at all!).

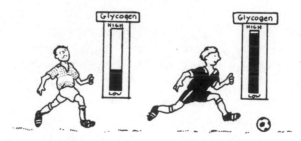

In summary, low glycogen stores lead to:

- early fatigue
- reduced training intensity
- reduced training gains
- poor performance
- increased injury risk
- slower recovery
- over training ('burnout') symptoms, if chronic.

How long does it take to refuel my glycogen stores after exercise?

The length of time that it takes to refuel depends on three main factors.

◆ How depleted your glycogen stores are after exercise.
◆ The amount and the timing of carbohydrate you eat.
◆ Your training experience and fitness level.

◆ Depletion

The more depleted your glycogen stores, the longer it will take you to refuel, just as it takes longer to refill an empty fuel tank than one that is half full. This, in turn, depends on the intensity and duration of your workout.

The higher the *intensity*, the more glycogen you use. For example, if you concentrate on fast, explosive activities (such as sprints, jumps or lifts) or high intensity aerobic activities (e.g. running), you will deplete your glycogen stores far more than for low intensity activities (e.g. walking, slow swimming) of equal duration.

The *duration* of your workout also has a bearing on the amount of glycogen you use. For example, if you run for one hour, you will use up more glycogen than if you run at the same speed for half an hour. If you complete 10 sets of shoulder presses in the gym, you will use more glycogen from your shoulder muscles than if you had completed only five sets at the same weight. Therefore, you need to allow more time to refuel after high intensity or long workouts.

◆ Carbohydrate intake

The higher your carbohydrate intake, the faster you can refuel your glycogen stores. Figure 1 shows how glycogen storage increases with carbohydrate intake.

This is particularly important if you train on a daily basis. Figure 2 shows the results of a study in which cyclists were given either a high (70%) carbohydrate diet or a low (40%) carbohydrate diet. Those with a high carbohydrate intake were able to refuel fully between daily training sessions, while those with a low intake could not.

Therefore, if you wish to train daily or every other day, make sure that you consume enough carbohydrate. If not, you will be

Figure 1: *Glycogen storage depends on carbohydrate intake*

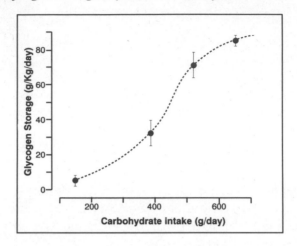

Figure 2: *A low carbohydrate intake results in poor refuelling*

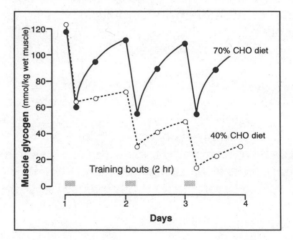

unable to train as hard or as long, you will suffer fatigue sooner and achieve smaller training gains.

◆ Training experience

Efficiency in refuelling improves automatically with training experience and raised fitness levels. Thus, it takes a beginner longer to replace his glycogen stores than an experienced athlete eating the same amount of carbohydrate. That's why élite sportspeople are able to train almost every day while beginners cannot and should not!

Another adaptation to training is an increase in your glycogen storing capacity, perhaps as much as 20%. This is an obvious advantage for training and competition. It is like upgrading from a 1l saloon car to a 3l sports car.

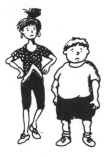

How much carbohydrate should I eat?

The consensus recommendation from the International Conference on Foods, Nutrition and Performance (1991) is a diet containing 60–70% energy from carbohydrate.

You can work out your carbohydrate intake in two ways.

1 From your energy intake

Calculate your energy (calorie) needs either by estimating from Tables 3 and 7 in Chapter 8 or by calculating your actual energy intake over three typical days, using food tables. Then multiply your energy intake by 60%, and divide by 4 to give you your recommended carbohydrate intake in grammes.

Example:

Energy intake = 3000 kcal

Energy from carbohydrate = 3000 × 60% = 1800

g carbohydrate = 1800 ÷ 4 = 450g

2 From your body weight and activity level

Calculate your activity level using the chart on page 36, then multiply this by your weight in kilogrammes.

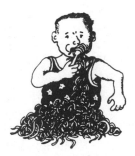

Table 1: *Daily carbohydrate requirements*

Activity level*	g carbohydrate/kg/day
Light (< 1h/day)	4–5
Light-moderate (approx. 1h/day)	5–6
Moderate (1–2h/day)	6–7
Moderate-heavy (2–4h/day)	7–8
Heavy (> 4h/day)	8–10

* Number of hours of medium intensity exercise or sport

Example:
If you weigh 80 kg and are moderately active (1 hour exercise per day)
Carbohydrate requirement = 80 × 6 = 480 g/day

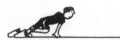

Use Tables 1, 2 and 3 to help you achieve your recommended carbohydrate intake. Most athletes find it useful to plan their meals and snacks in 50 g carbohydrate portions. For example, 10 portions of foods from Table 2 would give you approximately 500 g carbohydrate.

Table 2: *Food portions containing 50 g carbohydrate*

3 slices bread or toast
1 banana sandwich (2 slices bread + 1 banana)
Medium (2 oz) bowl breakfast cereal with ¼ pint low fat milk
Medium (6 oz) baked potato with 5 oz baked beans
7 oz cooked pasta
6 oz cooked rice
3 oz raisins/dates
2–3 dried fruit bars
1 pint isotonic sports drink
2–3 bananas
3–4 apples
5 cartons plain/low calorie yogurt
2 pints milk
11 oz cooked beans

Table 3: The carbohydrate and calorie content of various foods

Food	Portion	Carbohydrate (g)	Calories
Fruit			
Apple	1	10	39
Orange	1	10	42
Banana	1	19	79
Orange juice	150 ml	14	57
Raisins	30 g	19	75
Cereal			
Wholemeal bread	38 g (1 slice)	16	82
White bread	35 g (1 slice)	17	82
Spaghetti	75 g	56	257
Rice	50 g	43	181
Weetabix	2	30	136
Oats	30 g	20	113
Chapati (without fat)	55 g	24	111
Noodles (boiled)	150 g	19	93
Muesli (no added sugar)	40 g	27	146
Vegetables			
Potato (baked)	160 g	29	123
Sweet potato (boiled)	160 g	33	134
Sweetcorn	125 g	25	139
Baked beans	135 g	20	109
Red kidney beans (tinned)	200 g	36	200
Red lentils (boiled)	200 g	35	200
Cakes, biscuits and confectionery			
Sponge cake	65 g (1 slice)	42	196
Digestive biscuit	1	10	71
Honey	20 g (2 tsp)	15	58
Milk chocolate	50 g	30	265
Fruit cake	90 g (1 slice)	52	318
Currant bun	1	32	178

Food	Portion	Carbohydrate (g)	Calories
Puddings			
Apple crumble	170 g (1 portion)	62	352
Bread and butter pudding	170 g (1 portion)	30	272
Jelly	200 g (1 portion)	30	122
Dairy products			
Semi-skimmed milk	150 ml	7.3	67
Fruit yoghurt	150 g (1 pot)	26.9	135

How should I plan my meals?

In practice, you should base all your meals and snacks around foods which are high in carbohydrates. When planning a meal think *first* of a high carbohydrate food (such as bread or potatoes), and *then* work out what other foods to eat with it. For example, for lunch you may decide to have a potato based meal. So help yourself to a large baked potato (or two), and then add perhaps some tuna or cottage cheese, and lots of salad.

You may decide to have a pasta based meal in the evening. Make sure you have a large portion of pasta, and then add perhaps a tomato and vegetable sauce with some parmesan cheese.

The main rule when planning meals is always to include plenty of carbohydrate. Remember, if you do not eat enough carbohydrate, it will take you longer to refuel. Studies examining the differences in muscle glycogen levels after two days on a high carbohydrate diet, compared with two days on a low carbohydrate diet, show that muscle glycogen stores are not replenished after two days on a low carbohydrate diet.

How long should I rest between workouts?

In order to perform well, you have to leave enough time between training sessions to refill your glycogen stores. You must also eat a high carbohydrate diet, vary the intensity of training sessions, and allow yourself enough rest days.

If you have severely depleted your glycogen stores after a hard training session, you cannot expect to train hard again using the same muscles the following day. You need to allow more time to put the glycogen back. On the other hand, you may be able to do some light training as this will not tax the remaining glycogen stores. Better still, you may be able to do another form of training that exercises *different* muscle groups.

For example, if you work your legs muscles very hard on a Monday during a long cycle ride, multiple sprints or some heavy gym training, they will be very depleted. They will need several days (two to six, depending on how hard you have worked and how fit you are) to refuel completely. On Tuesday you could go on a short, gentle cycle ride, play tennis, or train a different muscle group (e.g. chest or arms) in the gym, or take a rest altogether.

If you attempt Monday's hard leg workout again on Tuesday, you will soon regret it! The exercises will feel extremely difficult to perform; you will not be able to work at the same intensity, or keep going for as long. You will also not be able to cycle as fast or as far; to sprint as fast or as many times; or to lift as many heavy weights in the gym for as many repetitions or sets.

In other words, you have to allow sufficient time for your muscles to recover and refuel between training sessions. Alternate heavy and light workouts, exercise different muscle groups, or take a complete rest between hard workouts.

If you have ever begun a training session with your legs feeling like hollow tubes, or had no power or strength during a workout, you now know why! These symptoms are a result of failure to refill your glycogen stores sufficiently.

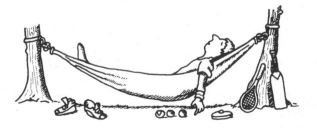

So, make sure that you start refuelling as soon as possible after your workout. Eat plenty of high carbohydrate foods (*see* page 37) at regular intervals, and do not attempt the same heavy training session until you feel that your muscles are sufficiently refuelled.

When is the best time to refuel?

The best time to start refuelling is as soon as possible after exercise, as glycogen storage is faster during the two hours immediately afterwards. Research has shown that muscle glycogen manufacture increases from the normal 5% to 7–8% per hour. Therefore, eating carbohydrate during this time allows you to refuel and recover faster before your next workout.

Aim to eat at least 1 g carbohydrate/kg body weight in this post exercise period. For example, if you weigh 80 kg, aim to eat around 80 g carbohydrate (e.g. ½ pint isotonic drink and one banana sandwich). You should have a minimum of 50 g carbohydrate. Even if you finish training late in the evening, you still need to start the refuelling process, so do not go to bed on an empty stomach! See Chapter 11 for ideas on suitable late evening snacks.

For efficient glycogen refuelling, you should continue to eat at least 50 g carbohydrate every two hours either in solid or liquid form. Therefore, plan your meals and snacks at frequent and regular intervals. If you leave long gaps without eating, glycogen storage and recovery will be slower. Similarly, if you eat most of your carbohydrate in just one or two large meals, storage will be less efficient and some of the carbohydrate may be converted into body fat.

Eating carbohydrates after exercise

In a recent study, athletes were given a carbohydrate drink either immediately after or two hours after exercise [1]. Glycogen storage during the first two hours following exercise turned out to be about three times faster in the athletes who had consumed carbohydrates straight away than it was in those who had, as yet, drunk nothing. Although glycogen manufacture speeded up when this second group of athletes had their carbohydrate drink (two hours after exercise), their overall rate of glycogen manufacture still turned out to be 45% slower than the first group in the four hours after exercise.

If you delay eating carbohydrate after exercise, glycogen manufacture will be slower and it will take longer to refuel.

1 Ivy *et al* (1988). *Muscle glycogen synthesis after exercise: effect of time on carbohydrate ingestion.* J Appl Physiol 64, 1480–1485.

Should I eat before exercise?

Many people wrongly believe that they should avoid sugars and other simple carbohydrates before exercise as these might trigger a surge of insulin and hypoglycaemia (low blood sugar). In fact, pre-exercise carbohydrate can help you to maintain higher blood sugar levels, delay fatigue, improve endurance and therefore help you to train harder for longer.

In an experiment at Cornell University, triathletes who ate 2–3 bananas immediately before a cycle trial were able to keep going 16–18 minutes longer than those who ate nothing. When researchers at Ohio State University gave cyclists a carbohydrate (sugar) drink one hour before a time trial, performance times improved by 12½% compared with those who drank a placebo. A study of sedentary men carried out in 1995 at the University of Massachusetts found that eating a confectionery bar before exercise did not adversely affect performance or result in hypoglycaemia.

Far from triggering a surge of insulin, exercise actually suppresses it by stimulating the production of adrenaline and other hormones which reduce insulin production, allowing blood sugar levels to be maintained longer. This is certainly an advantage: muscle glycogen may be spared, fatigue delayed and performance improved.

In practice, have approximately 50 g carbohydrate 5–30 minutes before you exercise, although you should leave at least two hours after your last meal. Experiment with different amounts of carbohydrate at different time intervals before exercise to find the strategy that suits you best.

Table 4: Suitable pre- or post-exercise snacks supplying 50 g carbohydrate

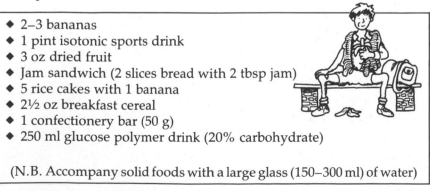

◆ 2–3 bananas
◆ 1 pint isotonic sports drink
◆ 3 oz dried fruit
◆ Jam sandwich (2 slices bread with 2 tbsp jam)
◆ 5 rice cakes with 1 banana
◆ 2½ oz breakfast cereal
◆ 1 confectionery bar (50 g)
◆ 250 ml glucose polymer drink (20% carbohydrate)

(N.B. Accompany solid foods with a large glass (150–300 ml) of water)

What is the difference between simple and complex carbohydrates?

Carbohydrates are sometimes divided into two categories: *simple* (sugars) and *complex* (starches and fibres). These terms refer to the number of sugar units in the molecule.

Simple carbohydrates are very small molecules consisting of one or two sugar units. They include glucose (dextrose), fructose (fruit sugar), sucrose (table sugar, which comprises a glucose and fructose molecule joined together) and lactose (milk sugar, which comprises a glucose and galactose molecule joined together).

Complex carbohydrates are very much larger molecules, consisting of thousands of sugar units (mostly glucose) joined together.

Between the simple and complex carbohydrates, although much closer to the former, are glucose polymers. These are man-made carbohydrates derived from the partial breakdown of corn starch, and consist of up to 20 sugar units.

Table 5: *Carbohydrate categories of various foods*

High in simple carbohydrates	High in complex carbohydrates	A mixture of simple and complex carbohydrates
Sugar (white and brown)	Flour (brown and white)	Cakes
Jam, honey and other preserves	Bread (all types)	Biscuits
Fruit (fresh, dried, tinned)	Pasta	Breakfast cereals (sweetened)
Yoghurt	Rice	Puddings
Fromage frais	Noodles	Sweet pastries, pies, flans
Ice cream	Oats	Cheesecake
Jelly	Other grains	Bananas
Confectionery	Breakfast cereals (unsweetened)	
Milk	Pulses (beans, lentils, peas)	
Soft drinks	Potatoes, yams, sweet potatoes, eddoes	
	Plantains (green bananas)	
	Parsnips	
	Sweetcorn	

In practice, many foods contain a mixture of both simple and complex carbohydrates. For example, biscuits and cakes contain flour (complex) and sugar (simple). Bananas contain a mixture of sugars and starches, depending on their degree of ripeness.

Which type of carbohydrate is best?

One type is not necessarily any healthier than the other. During digestion all carbohydrates are broken down into simple sugars and can equally well be converted into glycogen. So, from a physiological point of view, you can fuel muscles with either type. That's why this classification of carbohydrates into simple and complex is sometimes confusing and misleading for athletes.

What's more, different carbohydrate foods are suitable for different circumstances. There are three main things to consider.

♦ The nutritional package
♦ The glycaemic index
♦ The bulk.

1 The nutritional package

Carbohydrate foods that contain a range of other nutrients should comprise the main part of your daily diet. In general, foods rich in complex carbohydrates, e.g. bread and grains, and the naturally occurring simple carbohydrates, e.g. fruit and milk, have a better nutritional package than foods rich in refined simple carbohydrates, e.g. soft drinks and confectionery, (*see* Table 6).

In practice, therefore, aim to get most of your carbohydrates from foods providing a good nutrition package, i.e. bread, grains, cereals, starchy vegetables, pulses, fruit and dairy products. Less nutritious carbohydrate foods can still play a valuable role in your diet, as explained below. The occasional confectionery bar or cake will do you no harm; it is the overall balance of your diet that matters. It is important to enjoy your food without guilt.

2 The glycaemic index

The glycaemic index (GI) is a measure of the speed of carbohydrate absorption and rate of the resulting rise in blood sugar. It compares

43

Table 6: *Nutritional value of baked potato compared to a chocolate bar (equal number of calories)*

	Baked potato (8 oz/225 g)	Chocolate bar (1.5 oz/35 g)
Calories	154	154
Fat	< 1 g	7 g
Carbohydrate	36 g	23 g
Fibre	2.8 g	0 g
Sodium	14 mg	60 mg
Iron	0.8 mg	0.4 mg
Thiamin	0.42 mg	0.02 mg
Vitamin C	16 mg	0 mg

the rise in blood sugar produced after eating a food containing 50 g carbohydrate with a reference food (either glucose or white bread), which contains 50 g carbohydrate and has been assigned a value of 100. Therefore, the closer the GI of a food is to 100, the faster the rise in blood sugar produced. Most foods fall between 20 and 100, and are classified as having a high (60–100), medium (40–60) or low (< 40) GI (*see* Table 7, page 46).

The GI also takes into account the following factors which affect the rise in blood sugar.

◆ The presence of fibre (soluble fibre reduces the blood sugar rise).
◆ The presence of fat and protein (both reduce the blood sugar rise).
◆ The type of starch (e.g. starch in beans produces a slower blood sugar rise than starch in bread).
◆ Cooking and processing (cooked or processed starch produces a faster blood sugar rise).

Awareness of the GI of different foods is important to help you pick the right food for the right occasion. For example, sometimes there is a need to consume carbohydrates that can be quickly absorbed and transported to the muscles, such as immediately before exercise, during strenuous exercise and in the two hour period post exercise. Conversely, sometimes it is desirable to consume carbohydrates that are absorbed more slowly, e.g. in the 2–4 hour period

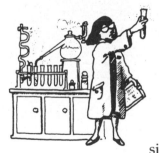

before exercise and the recovery period between workouts. Note, however, that the rate of absorption does not depend on the complexity of the carbohydrate. For example, potatoes produce a faster blood sugar rise than apples.

The GI is by no means a definitive guide. These values relate to the consumption of single foods on an empty stomach. Obviously, the GI of that food can be greatly modified if eaten with other foods as part of a meal. For example, bread eaten on its own has a high GI, but when eaten with cheese or baked beans, it will be lower. Therefore, use the GI values as a rough guide only.

3 Bulk

For those athletes with high energy and carbohydrate requirements, the sheer bulk of the diet can be a problem. Foods high in complex carbohydrates, particularly high fibre foods, can be very filling, making it difficult to eat enough food to satisfy your daily requirements. For example, if you need 3000 kcal per day you would need to eat the equivalent of 32 shredded wheats or 11 tins of baked beans to obtain the recommended intake of carbohydrate (450 g)!

While it is still important to eat plenty of wholegrain cereals, fruit and vegetables, you need to consider other ways of getting carbohydrate without the bulk. Less filling foods include white bread and dried fruit so it may be better to eat a mixture of wholemeal and white cereals, fresh and dried fruit, for example. Foods such as biscuits and carbohydrate drinks are also less bulky, yet high in carbohydrate. Use them to top up your carbohydrate intake, though, rather than relying on them for your major intake.

Should I eat carbohydrates during exercise?

If you are exercising for more than 60–90 minutes, extra carbohydrate during your workout may help delay fatigue and maintain your performance, particularly in the later stages. Researchers at California State University have also found that gains in muscle strength and size are greater if blood sugar levels are kept high during strength workouts. An intake of between 30 and 60 g

Table 7: *The Glycaemic Index of various foods (Glucose = 100)*

High (60–100)	GI	Moderate (40–60)	GI	Low (< 40)	GI
Cereals		*Cereals*		*Pulses*	
White bread	69	Wholemeal pasta	42	Butter beans	36
Wholemeal bread	72	White pasta	50	Baked beans	40
Brown rice	80	Oats	49	Haricot beans	31
White rice	82	Barley	22	Chick peas	36
				Lentils	29
				Kidney beans	29
				Soya beans	15
Breakfast cereals		*Breakfast cereals*			
Cornflakes	80	Porridge	54		
Muesli	66	All bran	51		
Shredded wheat	67				
Weetabix	75				
Fruit		*Fruit*		*Fruit*	
Raisins	64	Grapes	44	Apples	39
Bananas	62	Oranges	40	Cherries	23
				Plums	25
				Apricots	30
				Grapefruit	26
				Peaches	29
Vegetables		*Vegetables*		*Dairy products*	
Sweetcorn	59	Sweet potatoes	48	Milk	32
Parsnips	97	Crisps	51	Yoghurt	36
Baked potato	98	Yams	51	Ice cream	36
Carrots	92				
Other		*Other*		*Other*	
Biscuits	59	Oatmeal biscuits	54	Fructose	20
Chocolate bar	68	Sponge cake	46		
Honey	87				
Sucrose	59				
Glucose	100				
Orange cordial	66				

carbohydrate/hour, depending on your body weight and exercise intensity, is recommended by researchers at the University of Texas.

Any carbohydrate with a high glycaemic index would be suitable, but you may find liquids easier to consume than solids.

Isotonic sports drinks or carbohydrate (glucose polymer) drinks are usually helpful because they replace fluid loss and prevent dehydration as well as supplying carbohydrate.

If you can consume solids, choose high GI foods such as energy bars, bananas, dried fruit bars, or raisins and have a drink of water too. If you are competing in matches and tournaments (e.g. football, tennis), take suitable snacks and drinks for the intervals.

Researchers at Victoria University, Australia gave cyclists either 500 ml of a sports drink (5% carbohydrate), an energy bar plus water or just water. After two hours of exercise, blood sugar levels were maintained equally well with both the sports drink and the energy bar, but not with water.

Table 8: *What carbohydrate to eat and when?*

	Before exercise	During exercise	After exercise	Between workouts
How much?	50 g	30–60 g	1 g/kg body weight	60% of energy
Time period	5–30 min	Begin after 30 min; regular intervals	0–2 hours	Minimum 4–6 meals/snacks
GI	High	High	High	Low–moderate
Examples	◆ 2–3 bananas ◆ ½ pint isotonic sports drink & 1 banana ◆ 3 oz dried fruit ◆ Jam sandwich (2 slices bread with 2 tbsp jam) ◆ 1 confectionery bar	◆ 1l sports drink/ diluted squash (3–6%) ◆ Energy bar ◆ 2–3 bananas ◆ 2–3 oz dried fruit	◆ Banana sandwich ◆ 3 oz raisins ◆ 4–5 low fat biscuits ◆ 250 ml glucose polymer drink (20%) ◆ 8 oz potato	◆ Pasta with lentils/low fat cheese/ chicken/fish ◆ Rice with beans ◆ Noodles with tofu/ poultry/ seafood ◆ Beans on toast ◆ Potato with cottage cheese/tuna

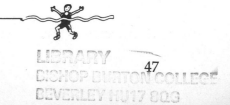

SUMMARY OF KEY POINTS

◆ For optimal training gains, ensure that muscle glycogen stores are fully restored between training sessions.

◆ The length of time taken to refuel glycogen stores between training sessions depends on the intensity and duration of exercise (i.e. the degree of depletion); the amount and timing of carbohydrate intake; and your fitness level.

◆ It takes longer to refuel following high intensity and/or prolonged exercise; on a low carbohydrate diet; and with lower fitness levels.

◆ The recommended carbohydrate intake for athletes and active people is 60–70% of total energy intake. In practice, most athletes need to consume 6–10 g carbohydrate/kg body weight/day.

◆ Glycogen refuelling is faster in the 2 hour period following exercise. A carbohydrate intake of at least 1 g/kg body weight is recommended during this time.

◆ For efficient refuelling, continue to consume a minimum of 50 g carbohydrate every 2 hours.

◆ Leave approximately 2–3 hours between your last meal and training. Consuming a further 50 g carbohydrate immediately before exercise may help maintain blood sugar levels, delay fatigue and improve performance.

◆ For strenuous exercise lasting more than 60–90 minutes, consuming 30–60 g carbohydrate (in liquid or solid form) during exercise can help maintain performance longer.

◆ The choice of which type of carbohydrate depends on its nutritional package, its glycaemic index (GI) and its bulk.

◆ The main part of the diet should comprise carbohydrate foods with a good overall nutritional package, e.g. bread and cereals, pulses, starchy vegetables, fruit and low fat dairy products.

◆ Carbohydrates with a high GI produce a fast rise in blood sugar and are therefore advantageous before, during and after exercise.

◆ Athletes with very high energy and carbohydrate requirements should include a mixture of high and low bulk carbohydrate foods in their diet in order to eat enough to satisfy their daily requirements.

3

Protein – the stronghold?

The importance of protein in athletic performance is one of the most hotly debated nutritional topics among scientists, coaches and sportspeople. Whether extra protein is needed or not has been contended ever since the time of the Ancient Greeks. It is tempting to think that a high protein intake helps to increase muscle size and strength, since protein is the major constituent of muscles. Is this wishful thinking or fact?

Until recently, nutritionists believed that sportspeople did not need more protein than sedentary people, and that eating more than the standard recommended daily intake was unlikely to produce any benefits.

However, research over the last ten years has cast doubt on this view. There are indications that the protein needs of strength and endurance athletes may be higher than it has always been believed.

This chapter will help to give you a fuller understanding of the role of protein during exercise, and enable you to work out how much you need. It will show how individual requirements depend on the sport concerned and the training programme, and also how they are related to carbo-hydrate intake. An example of a daily menu is given to show how to meet your own protein re-quirements, and to provide a basis for developing your own

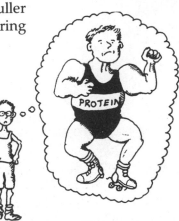

menu. This chapter also discusses the controversial issues of protein and amino acid supplementation.

Why do I need protein?

Protein is an important nutrient, because it makes up part of the structure of every cell in the body. About three-quarters of the dry weight of human muscle is protein. Structural tissues such as tendons, skin, hair and nails are also made of protein. Overall, it comprises about 20% of total body weight.

Protein is necessary for the growth and formation of new tissues, and also for repairing damaged tissues. A regular supply of protein is needed in your diet to compensate for the continual loss that occurs in the body. Proteins are constantly being broken down (catabolism) and built up again (anabolism) in every cell. Some of them are recycled, but there is always an overall loss. If you are involved in a strength sport, you will need a little extra to allow for new tissue growth.

Protein is also needed to make thousands of different enzymes in your body, as well as certain hormones such as insulin and adrenaline.

Figure 1: *Proteins are continually broken down and recycled*

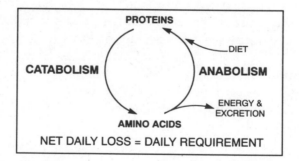

Does protein provide energy?

Protein may also be used as a fuel source, yielding 4 kcal/g (17 kJ/g), the same as carbohydrate. However, this is not its primary function since it is more difficult for the body to convert protein into energy than to use carbohydrate. Under normal circumstances, only very small quantities are broken down. However, when glycogen is in short supply (for example, during dieting or towards the end of a strenuous workout), increased quantities of protein are converted into energy, supplying up to 10% of the fuel mixture. This occurs at the expense of other tissues (mostly from muscles and, possibly, organs) and, over time, can lead to substantial losses of lean body mass. That is why training on a low carbohydrate diet produces few or no gains and is a common factor in the over training syndrome ('burnout').

What are proteins?

Proteins are made up of smaller units called amino acids. There are 20 different amino acids in all, and they can be combined in many ways to form hundreds of different proteins. Each protein consists of thousands of amino acids linked together.

When you eat a food containing protein, it is broken down in the digestive system into its constituent amino acids, then reassembled into the particular proteins that your body needs at the time (*see* fig. 2, below).

Figure 2: Digestion and absorption of protein

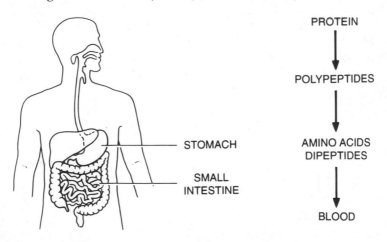

The body is capable of making 12 non essential (or dispensable) amino acids on its own (from intermediate products of carbohydrate or protein metabolism) if it needs to, but eight cannot be produced and must be supplied in the diet. They are called essential (or indispensable) amino acids.

In fact, strictly speaking, the body's requirement is for amino acids rather than protein.

How much protein do I need?

Protein needs are normally expressed per kg body weight, i.e. the larger you are, the greater your protein requirements. The Department of Health recommend 0.75 g/kg/day for sedentary adults, or a Reference Nutrient Intake (*see* page 67) of 55.5 g/day for an average man weighing 74 kg and 45 g/day for an average woman weighing 60 kg. Requirements increase during pregnancy and breastfeeding.

However, these recommendations do not take account of regular strenuous exercise, and studies have shown that sportspeople have increased needs. At the International Conference on Foods, Nutrition and Sports Performance in 1991, experts recommended that athletes should consume between 1.2 and 1.7 g/kg/day. The lower end of the range (1.2–1.4 g/kg) is more appropriate for endurance activities, while the upper end of the range (1.4–1.7 g/kg) is recommended for strength and power activities.

Thus, a distance runner weighing 70 kg will need 84–98 g/day. A sprinter or weightlifter with the same body weight will need 98–119 g/day. In practice, these protein intakes are not difficult to achieve if you are eating enough food to meet your energy and carbohydrate requirements. Protein intakes generally reflect total calorie intake, which is why the International Conference stated that protein should comprise 12–15% of total energy intake, the same as for sedentary people.

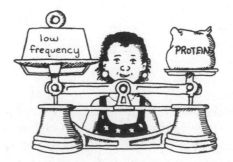

Table 1: *Amino Acids*

Essential	Non essential
Isoleucine	Alanine
Leucine	Arginine
Lysine	Asparagine
Methionine	Aspartic acid
Phenylalanine	Cysteine
Threonine	Glutamic acid
Tryptophan	Glutamine
Valine	Glycine
	Histidine*
	Proline
	Serine
	Tyrosine

* Histidine is essential for babies (not for adults)

How does exercise affect my protein requirement?

Studies have shown that exercise increases protein breakdown and, therefore, dietary requirement. The exact amount depends on the following factors.

◆ The type, intensity and frequency of your training.
◆ How long you have been training.
◆ Your calorie and carbohydrate intake.

1 Type, intensity and frequency of training

Evidence suggests that protein breakdown increases during and immediately after exercise, and that protein manufacture (anabolism) slows down at the same time. In other words, exercise causes an overall breakdown of protein, which ultimately affects the body's requirements. The longer you exercise, the more protein is broken down. For example, you would break down more proteins during a two hour run than a one hour run.

Intensity is also a crucial factor in determining protein needs. The more intense the exercise, the greater your protein breakdown and the greater your needs. Exercise seems to be a trigger in activating a particular enzyme that oxidises certain amino acids. The greater the stimulus, the greater the enzyme activation and protein breakdown.

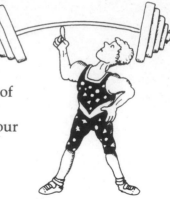

If you do not eat enough protein to compensate for the increased breakdown and/or if you train too frequently, this net loss of lean tissue will eventually affect your performance. Reduced muscle size and strength is one of the typical symptoms of overtraining.

If you train to increase muscle mass, your protein needs will be greater still. Extra protein will be needed not only to compensate for protein breakdown, caused by the intense training, but also for new protein to be made for muscle growth. Too small an intake may cause slower muscle growth or even muscle loss, despite hard training. However, in practice the body *adapts* to a regularly low intake of protein, and so progress can still be made. The body can also adapt to a consistently high protein intake.

You may eat considerably smaller amounts of protein than your training partner and follow the same training programme, but still have exactly the same muscle mass and strength level. This is because your body will have adapted to the lower intake over time. Even if you were to eat more protein, your muscle mass and strength would not necessarily increase.

It is important to realise that a high protein diet alone will not lead to any increase in strength or muscle size. It is only when it is combined with heavy resistance exercise that additional protein can cause this to happen.

2 Length of training

The protein needs of newcomers to exercise are different from those of sportspeople who have been training for some time. Recent studies have shown that beginners have higher requirements per kg/body weight than more experienced athletes. Initially, a beginner will experience an increase in protein needs due to increases in protein turnover (especially protein breakdown). After a few weeks of exercise, however, the body becomes accustomed to training and becomes more efficient at recycling proteins. Broken down proteins can be built up again from released amino acids, so there is less 'waste' than before. The body also becomes more efficient in conserving protein. The net result is a decrease in protein requirements. Some studies have shown that the requirements per kg of novice bodybuilders can be up to 40% higher than those of experienced bodybuilders.

Ultimately, however, people who exercise regularly still have higher protein needs per kg than sedentary people.

Figure 3: *Protein balance before/after training programme*

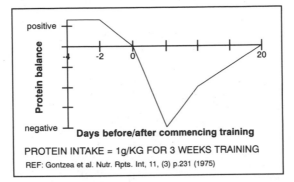

PROTEIN INTAKE = 1g/KG FOR 3 WEEKS TRAINING
REF: Gontzea et al. Nutr. Rpts. Int, 11, (3) p.231 (1975)

3 Diet

As we have already seen, if you do not consume enough calories to meet your needs, protein will be broken down for energy rather than being used for growth and repair. Satisfying energy requirements is the body's top priority.

This has implications if you are dieting – for example, if you are trying to make weight for competition. By cutting your energy and carbohydrate intake you will automatically increase your protein needs, so you should aim to maintain your carbohydrate intake. Choose low fat protein foods, such as skimmed milk, skinless chicken and pulses. In this way you can keep your fat intake low, while maintaining protein levels and reducing calories.

In Chapter 1 we saw how a low carbohydrate intake can lead to a rapid depletion of glycogen during exercise. This in turn causes increased protein breakdown to provide fuel for energy. Rapid fatigue and an unnecessary breakdown of tissue are the results.

Conversely, as carbohydrate intake increases, protein requirements decrease. Studies have shown that athletes in a positive energy balance (who eat more energy than they need) have smaller net losses of protein, and therefore smaller protein requirements. Sportspeople wishing to increase their muscle mass must therefore make sure that they are obtaining sufficient energy and carbohydrate, as well as sufficient protein, from their diet.

Are protein and glycogen related?

Although protein is not a major source of fuel during exercise, certain amino acids (e.g. leucine and lysine) can be broken down to provide energy when glycogen levels are low. This may be important in sports where the energy demand is high and prolonged, such as marathon running, weight training and sprint training.

However, when glycogen levels are high, there is far less chance that amino acids will be broken down. Glycogen, therefore, has a protein sparing effect. This means that if there is plenty of glycogen in an exercising muscle, the protein breakdown will be minimal. But when glycogen stores become depleted, protein breakdown increases, so it is important to start exercising with full glycogen stores. Not only will this help to delay fatigue, but it will also prevent excessive protein breakdown.

Protein breakdown

In one study, protein breakdown was measured in six athletes who exercised for one hour. The athletes were either following a low carbohydrate diet (to produce low glycogen stores) or a high carbohydrate diet (to increase glycogen stores). The protein breakdown was considerably higher in the athletes who exercised with low glycogen stores.

Do strength athletes need extra protein?

A number of recent studies involving sophisticated techniques for measuring changes in muscle size have suggested that high protein diets combined with heavy resistance training can enhance muscle strength and size.

For example, in one study [1] male athletes who consumed an extra 23 g protein per day during 12 weeks of strength training achieved significantly greater size gains than those who did not take extra protein. However, strength gains were similar in both groups.

In a study carried out at McMaster University [2], strength

1 W.R. Frontera *et al.*, Canadian Journal of Sports Sciences, 13(2), 1988.
2 M.A. Tarnopolsky *et al.*, Journal of Applied Physiology, 73(5), 1992.

athletes were given either a low protein (0.86 g/kg), medium protein (1.4 g/kg) or high protein (2.4 g/kg) diet for 13 days. The low protein diet, which is similar to the recommended diet for sedentary people, caused the athletes to lose body protein (muscle mass). However, both the medium and high protein diets resulted in an increased body protein content, i.e. their muscle mass increased. No further gains were made by increasing their intake from 1.4 g to 2.4 g/kg.

Thus, muscle mass gains do not increase in a linear fashion with increasing protein intake. Once an optimal intake has been reached, surplus protein is not converted into muscle.

In conclusion, the studies on strength athletes indicate that

Table 2: *The protein content of various foods*

FOOD	PROTEIN (g per portion)
Meat/Fish/Poultry	
Red meat (4 oz portion)	32
Chicken (6 oz portion)	38
White fish (6 oz portion)	30
Oily fish (6 oz portion)	30
Sausages (2)	15
Mince (4 oz)	25
Tinned tuna (4 oz)	25
Dairy Products and eggs	
Milk (½ pint)	10
Cottage cheese (4 oz)	15
Fromage frais (4 oz)	8
Cheddar cheese (2 oz)	14
Yoghurt (1 carton)	8
Eggs (2)	14
Pulses and nuts	
Kidney beans (8 oz boiled)	15
Baked beans (½ large tin)	10
Lentils (8 oz boiled)	15
Nuts (2 oz)	13
Cereals	
Bread (2 slices)	6
Pasta (6 oz boiled)	5
Rice (6 oz boiled)	4
Other	
Tofu (4 oz)	9

strength training increases protein requirements to approximately 1.4–1.7 g/kg/day.

How can I meet my protein needs?

For the majority of people, it is not difficult to meet protein needs from food alone, as it is found in a wide range of foods. Table 2 lists the protein content of a selection.

The usefulness of a particular protein is often measured by its biological value (**BV**), which indicates how closely matched the proportion of amino acids is to the body's requirements. It is a measure of the percentage of protein retained by the body for use in growth and tissue maintenance. Egg white, for example, has a BV of 100, which means it contains all the essential amino acids the body requires in closely matched proportions, so that virtually all of the food protein can be used for making new body proteins.

Other foods (mainly plant foods) contain significant amounts of protein, but are short of one or two essential amino acids (called limiting amino acids). These have a lower BV, but eating a mixture of these during the day is just as good as eating proteins with a high BV. By eating a mixture of foods with a low BV, the shortfall of amino acids in one is complemented by higher amounts in the other, so the resulting amino acid intake increases the overall BV. This is called protein complementation. In other words, it is not essential to obtain your protein needs purely from high BV sources; a variety of both low and high BV protein foods is a healthy way to meet your requirements.

For example, lysine is a limiting amino acid in cereals and methionine is a limiting amino acid in beans. Put the two foods together, as in baked beans on toast, and the two foods complement each other, so that you end up with a well balanced mixture of amino acids.

Examples of other suitable combinations include:

- porridge (cereal and milk)
- red kidney beans and rice (pulses and cereal)
- peanut butter sandwich (nuts and cereal)
- lentil soup with roll (pulses and cereal)
- chilli con carne (pulses and meat)
- breakfast cereal and milk (cereal and milk).

Table 3: *The BV content of various foods*

Foods with a high BV	Foods with a low BV
Milk, cheese, yoghurt Meat, fish, poultry Eggs Soya products (soya beans/milk/ textured vegetable protein/tofu)	Pulses – beans, lentils, peas Bread, cereals, grains Nuts and seeds

How can I make sure that my diet covers my protein needs?

Use Table 2 to help you estimate your current protein intake. Table 4 gives an example of a daily menu which meets the protein requirements of an athlete weighing 70 kg. It provides approximately 3000 kcal and 120 g protein. Use this as a basis for developing your own daily menu.

Table 4: *Sample eating plan providing approx. 3000 calories, 120 g protein*

Breakfast	3 oz (75 g) cereal with ½ pint (300 ml) milk 2 slices toast and marmalade 1 glass fruit juice
Snack	Tuna sandwich (2 slices bread) 2 pieces fruit
Lunch	2 jacket potatoes with 8 oz (225 g) baked beans Salad 1–2 pieces fruit with one yoghurt
Snack	6 rice cakes/crackers 1 banana
Dinner	6 oz (175 g) pasta with tomato/vegetable sauce 3 oz (75 g) chicken Vegetables 1 piece fruit and 1 yoghurt
Snack	2 slices toast 2 pieces fruit

Are high protein foods also high in fat?

Some high protein foods, such as full fat dairy products, red meat and meat products, also contain quite a high proportion of fat. Obviously, if these make up a large part of your diet, this can result in a high overall fat intake, which is disadvantageous for health and performance.

You can still maintain an adequate protein intake and consume a low to moderate fat diet by choosing reduced fat alternatives of your usual foods (*see* Table 5).

Table 5: *Reduced fat alternatives of various foods*

Food	Lower fat alternatives
Red meat (regular cut)	Lean cut (fat trimmed) Chicken/turkey (without skin)
Full fat milk	Semi-skimmed or skimmed milk
Hard cheese	Reduced fat hard cheese Low fat soft cheeses, e.g. cottage cheese, fromage frais, quark

Plant foods that provide protein, such as cereals and pulses, are very low in fat, so try to eat them more often. For example, use beans or lentils to replace some or all of the meat in casseroles, stews and pies. When cooking meat or poultry, use methods which do not involve the addition of fat and oil. For example, grill, bake, poach, boil, barbecue or microwave instead of frying. Add herbs, spices and other flavouring ingredients to enhance the taste. For more recipe ideas, *see* Chapter 12.

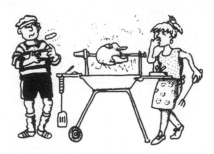

Is too much protein harmful?

Consuming more protein than you need offers no advantage in terms of health or physical performance. Extra protein is not converted into muscle and does not cause further increases in muscle size, strength or stamina.

The amino group of protein that contains nitrogen is converted in the liver into a substance called *urea*. This is then passed to the kidneys and excreted in the urine. The remainder of the protein is converted into glucose and used as an energy substrate. It may either be used as fuel immediately or stored – usually as glycogen. If you are already eating enough carbohydrate and therefore refilling your glycogen stores, excess glucose may be converted into fat. However, recent studies have shown that eating protein increases the metabolic rate, so a significant proportion of the protein calories are oxidised and given off as heat. Thus, a slight excess of protein is unlikely to be converted into fat.

It was once thought that excess protein might cause liver or kidney damage by placing undue stress on these organs. However, this has never been demonstrated in healthy people and so remains only a theoretical possibility.

It has also been claimed that eating too much protein leads to dehydration because extra water is drawn from the body's fluids to dilute and excrete the increased quantities of urea. This is unlikely to be a problem if you drink enough fluids.

In his work reported in *Nutrition Abstracts and Reviews* (54, 447–59, 1984), Yuen D. *et al.* suggested there is some evidence that high protein diets can cause an excessive excretion of calcium, increasing the risk of osteoporosis.

In conclusion, however, eating too much protein is unlikely to be harmful, but offers no advantage in terms of performance or muscle size either.

Is it a good idea to take protein supplements?

Most protein supplements consist of powdered milk and/or egg protein or soya, often with the addition of other ingredients, such as glucose polymers, amino acids, vitamins, minerals and various substances claiming to increase growth.

Despite the powerful advertising, protein based supplements do not in themselves encourage increases in muscle growth, strength or endurance. They may contribute to your daily protein intake, but do not expect to gain extra muscle simply by taking them! Even the added 'growth promoting' substances have no proven benefit (*see* Chapter 5: Other pills and potions).

You can meet your protein requirements from food, providing you plan your diet sensibly. One pint of milk (any type), for example, provides roughly the same amount of protein as one serving of a standard protein supplement – but for considerably less money! Supplements may be regarded as an alternative to food, not as a substitute.

The only case where supplements may be useful is for people with very high calorie and protein requirements, who would otherwise find it difficult to eat enough food to fulfil these. As an addition to meals, they provide a low bulk way of consuming extra calories, protein and other nutrients. In these cases, it is best to choose a supplement which provides a good balance of carbohydrate, protein, vitamins and minerals. Consume the supplement in addition to your meals, not in place of them.

Remember that protein over and above your requirements will not be turned into muscle!

Should I take amino acid supplements?

Many athletes believe that taking amino acid supplements increases their strength, muscle mass or stamina. Manufacturers claim the supplements are useful because they do not need to be digested and are therefore absorbed faster. Unfortunately, there is no evidence that faster absorption of amino acids is beneficial because it takes hours – not minutes – to build new muscle proteins!

Another claim is that a greater percentage of amino acids is absorbed from supplements than from food. In fact, more than 80–90% of amino acids from food is utilised by the body anyway. Bear in mind that one amino acid tablet provides only 1 g or less whereas a tuna or cottage cheese sandwich provides around 20 g! Relatively large amounts would need to be taken to have a significant impact on your total daily amino acid (protein) intake – and this would work out very expensive!

It appears, therefore, that there are no advantages in taking amino acid supplements.

Do certain amino acid supplements really promote growth hormone release?

It has been claimed that certain combinations of amino acids – ornithine/arginine/lysine – increase the body's own production of the growth hormone, which stimulates muscle growth and fat oxidation. Manufacturers instruct athletes to take them before sleeping and prior to training. However, this is not based on any valid scientific research – early studies using massive injected doses have not been validated. Oral supplements have no effect on growth hormone levels.

In a study carried out at the University of Pittsburgh, eight male athletes completed two weight training sessions, one with and one without supplements. Both workouts produced an equal increase in growth hormone output.

Exercise and sleep are natural promoters of growth hormone release – so hard training and plenty of rest will benefit your performance much more than amino acid supplements.

Do 'branch chain' amino acid supplements work?

Branched amino acids include the three amino acids with a branched geometrical configuration: leucine, valine and iso-leucine. They make up about 70% of muscle proteins and are broken down in increased quantities during intense prolonged exercise as glycogen becomes depleted. Some manufacturers claim that supplementing these particular amino acids before, during and after intense exercise may reduce or offset muscle protein breakdown. However, there is little evidence that supplements have a significant effect.

For example, in a study carried out at the University of Limburg in 1994, 10 athletes were given either a sugar/electrolyte sports drink with added branched chain amino acids or just the sports drink on its own. They were then instructed to cycle to the point of exhaustion. All reached this point at the same time, so researchers concluded that the branched chain amino acids had no effect on performance or endurance.

Taking extra carbohydrate during exercise seems to be the best way to offset protein breakdown.

SUMMARY OF KEY POINTS

- Proteins make up part of the structure of every cell in the body, including about three quarters of the dry weight of muscle; they also form enzymes and hormones.
- Proteins are continually broken down into amino acids and recycled as new proteins or energy substrates. Some protein is therefore lost every day and must be replaced in the diet.
- More protein is broken down to provide energy when glycogen is in short supply, e.g. during dieting or prolonged intense exercise.
- Exercise increases protein breakdown and therefore dietary requirements. The exact amount depends on the type, frequency, duration and intensity of exercise; your fitness level; and your energy and carbohydrate intake.
- The protein needs of athletes are greater than those of sedentary people. An intake between 1.2 and 1.7 g/kg body weight/day, equivalent to 12–15% energy intake, is recommended.
- Strength training increases protein needs more than aerobic training. An intake of 1.4–1.7 g/kg is recommended for strength athletes, and an intake of 1.2–1.4 g/kg for endurance athletes.
- Athletes should be able to meet their increased protein needs from a balanced diet that is meeting their energy needs.
- High protein intakes, surplus to requirements, do not enhance muscle strength, size or mass and therefore offer no advantage.
- Protein supplements are unnecessary for most athletes and do not automatically enhance performance or strength. They may be useful if energy and protein requirements cannot be met from food alone.
- There is no evidence to support the claims for amino acid supplements.

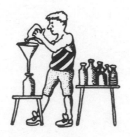

CHAPTER

4

Vitamins, minerals and supplements

Vitamins and minerals are often equated with vitality, energy and strength. Many people think of them as health enhancers, a plentiful supply being the secret to a long and healthy life.

In fact, vitamins and minerals do not in themselves provide any energy at all. Nor does an abundant supply automatically guarantee bounce and vigour or optimal health.

The truth is that vitamins and minerals are needed in certain quantities for good health, as well as for peak physical performance. However, it is the *balance* of vitamins and minerals in the diet that is most important.

For sportspeople, it is tempting to think that extra vitamins lead to better performance. Because a small amount is 'good for us', more would surely be better. Or would it?

This chapter explains what vitamins and minerals do, where they come from, and how exercise affects requirements. Do athletes need extra amounts; and should they take supplements?

This chapter also examines the claims made by supplement manufacturers. (In most cases claims are implied rather than stated because, by law, supplement manufacturers cannot make direct medical claims or state that their products will benefit athletic performance.) Only claims relevant to sports performance are considered here.

What are vitamins?

Vitamins are required in tiny amounts for growth, health and physical well-being. Many form the essential parts of enzyme systems, which are involved in energy production and exercise performance. Others are involved in the functioning of the immune system, the hormonal system and the nervous system.

Our bodies are unable to make vitamins, so they must be supplied in our diet.

What are minerals?

Minerals are inorganic elements that have many regulatory and structural roles in the body. Some (such as calcium and phosphorus) form part of the structure of bones and teeth. Others are involved in controlling the fluid balance in tissues, muscle contraction, nerve function, enzyme secretion and the formation of red blood cells. Like vitamins, they cannot be made in the body and must be obtained in the diet.

How much do I need?

Everyone has different nutritional requirements. These vary according to age, size, activity and individual body chemistry. It is, therefore, impossible to state an intake that would be right for everyone. To find out your exact requirements you would have to undergo a series of biochemical and physiological tests.

However, scientists have studied groups of people with similar characteristics, such as age and physical activity, and have come up with some estimates of requirements. Until recently these were called Recommended Daily Amounts (RDAs) – you may have noticed them on food labels. RDAs have recently been revised, and new standards, called Dietary Reference Values (DRVs) have now been set by the Committee on Medical Aspects of Food Policy (COMA). This is an umbrella term used to cover all the values.

What are dietary reference values?

Three values have been set for each nutrient:

1 **The Estimated Average Requirement (EAR)** is the amount of a nutrient needed by an average person, so many people will need more or less.

2 **The Reference Nutrient Intake (RNI)** is the amount of a nutrient that should cover the needs of 97% of the population. It is more than most people require, and only a very few people (3%) will exceed it.
3 **The Lower Reference Nutrient Intake (LRNI)** is for a small number of people who have low needs (about 3% of the population). Most people will need more than this amount.

In practice, most people are somewhere in the middle. Athletes and sportspeople probably approach the upper limits.

How are DRVs set?

It is not easy to set a DRV. First of all, scientists have to work out what is the *minimum* amount of a particular nutrient that a person needs to be healthy. Once this has been established, scientists usually add on a safety margin, to take account of individual variations. No two people will have exactly the same requirement. Next, a *storage requirement* is assessed. This allows for a small reserve of the nutrient to be kept in the body.

Unfortunately, scientific evidence of human vitamin and mineral requirements is fairly scanty and contradictory. A lot of scientific guesswork is inevitably involved, and results are often extrapolated from animal studies.

In practice, DRVs are arrived at through a compromise between selected scientific data and good judgement. They vary from country to country and are always open to debate.

Should I plan my diet around the Reference Nutrient Intake?

The RNI is not a target intake to aim for – it is only a guideline. It should cover the needs of most people but, of course, it is possible that some athletes may need more than the RNI, due to their higher energy expenditure.

In practice, if you are getting the RNI for a particular nutrient, you are very likely to be meeting your needs. If you are eating substantially and consistently less than the RNI, you may be lacking in that nutrient.

Can a balanced diet provide all the vitamins and minerals I need?

In theory you should be able to get all the vitamins and minerals you need from a well planned diet. This should include a wide variety of foods from each of the main food groups in roughly the proportions recommended by the Department of Health (*see* below). In other words, cereals, vegetables and fruit should make up the bulk of your diet, followed by dairy products, meat/ vegetarian alternatives, oils and fats. Obviously, each food group supplies a different balance of nutrients, which is why it is important to plan your diet well.

If you exercise regularly and eat in accordance with your appetite (i.e. you are not dieting), you should be eating more food than the average sedentary person. This means you should automatically achieve a higher vitamin and mineral intake, providing you are not simply filling up on sugary fatty foods with a low nutrient density!

However, in practice many people do not plan their diets well or they restrict their calorie intake so it can be difficult to obtain sufficient amounts of vitamins and minerals from food. Vitamin losses also occur during food processing, preparation and cooking, thus further reducing your actual intake.

Table 1: *Achieving a balanced diet**

Foods	Portions/Day
Cereals and starchy vegetables	5–11
Fruit and vegetables	> 5
Milk and dairy products	2–3
Meat, fish and vegetarian alternatives	2–3
Oils and fats	0–3

* National Food Guide, DoH, 1994

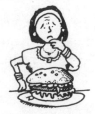

Can vitamin and mineral supplements improve your performance?

Many studies have been carried out over the years using varying doses of supplements. In the vast majority of cases, scientists have been unable to measure significant improvements in performance in healthy athletes. Where a beneficial effect has been observed, for example increasing endurance, this has tended to be in athletes with a sub-optimal vitamin or mineral status to start with. Taking supplements simply restored the athletes' nutrient stores to 'normal' levels. However, once this had been reached, no further improvements in performance were measured.

In other words, low body stores or deficient intakes can adversely affect your performance, but vitamin and mineral supplements taken in excess of your requirements will not necessarily produce a further improvement in performance. More does not mean better! Most are unlikely to be of benefit if you are eating a well balanced diet.

When may supplements be useful?

Eating a balanced diet may not always be easy in practice, particularly if you travel a lot, work shifts or long hours, train at irregular times, eat on the run or are unable to purchase and prepare your own meals. Planning and eating a well balanced diet requires considerably more effort under these circumstances, so you may not be getting all the vitamins and minerals you need. A deficient intake is also likely if you are on a restricted diet (e.g., eating less than 2000 calories a day for a period of time or excluding a food group from your regular diet).

A number of surveys have shown that many sportspeople do not achieve an adequate intake of vitamins and minerals from their diet. Female athletes in particular tend to have lower intakes of iron, calcium and some of the B vitamins. You may therefore wish to consider supplements as a form of insurance, but it is always best to get your vitamins and minerals from your diet rather than relying on supplements.

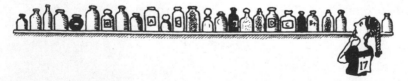

Who may benefit from taking supplements?

Obviously, supplements are not a substitute for poor or lazy eating habits. If you think you may be lacking in vitamins and minerals, try to adjust your diet to include more vitamin and mineral rich foods.

As a temporary measure, you may benefit from taking supplements if:

◆ you have erratic eating habits
◆ you eat less than 2000 kcal a day
◆ you are pregnant (folic acid)
◆ you eat out a lot/rely on fast foods
◆ you are a vegan (vitamin B12)
◆ you are anaemic
◆ you have a major food allergy or intolerance (e.g. milk)
◆ you are a heavy smoker or drinker
◆ you are ill or convalescing.

Does exercise increase my requirements?

Regular intense exercise increases your requirements for a number of vitamins and minerals, particularly those involved in energy metabolism (e.g. B vitamins), tissue growth and repair (e.g. vitamin A, zinc), red blood cell manufacture (e.g. iron) and free radical defence (e.g. beta-carotene, vitamins C and E). However, you should be able to meet these needs by a corresponding increase in your food intake. There is a direct relationship between food intake and vitamin/mineral intake – the more you eat, the more vitamins and minerals you get.

Will supplements improve my physical performance?

While a deficiency will adversely affect your performance, there is no strong evidence that taking supplements in excess of your requirements will improve it. To find out if your diet is deficient in any nutrient, you should consult a qualified nutritionist (look for the initials BSc or SRD) for a dietary analysis. He or she will then be able to advise you about your diet and supplementation, if necessary.

Can supplements be harmful?

Some vitamins and minerals taken in high doses can be toxic. The fat soluble vitamins A and D, vitamin B6, as well as several minerals, can be stored in organs and fatty tissues (e.g. the liver, adipose tissue) and, therefore, accumulate over time.

Excess vitamin A can cause nausea, skin changes such as flakiness, liver damage and birth defects in unborn babies. Pregnant women are advised to avoid vitamin A supplements, fish liver oils and concentrated food sources of vitamin A such as liver and liver paté. Too much vitamin D from supplements can cause high blood pressure and kidney stones. Excessive doses of vitamin B6 may lead to numbness, persistent pins and needles and unsteadiness (a type of neuropathy). High doses of iron can cause constipation and discomfort through an upset or bloated stomach.

Vitamin C and the B vitamins are water soluble and are therefore not stored in the body. Excessive intakes are excreted from the body in the urine, although extremely high intakes from supplements may have minor adverse effects (*see* pages 80–87).

Vitamin E, on the other hand, is a fat soluble vitamin which appears to be safe even at doses 10–100 times the recommended intake. There is evidence that supplements of up to 80 mg/day may be beneficial in preventing heart disease.

Except perhaps in the case of liver (owing to modern animal feeding practices), it is almost impossible to overdose on vitamins and minerals from food. Problems are more likely to arise from the indiscriminate use of supplements, so always follow the guidelines on the label or the advice of a nutritionist, and never take more than 10 times the RDA of any of the fat soluble vitamins and minerals.

Can supplements cause imbalances?

Taking single vitamins or minerals can easily lead to imbalances and deficiencies. Many interact with each other, competing for absorption, enhancing or impairing each other's functions. For example, iron, zinc and calcium share the same absorption and transport system, so taking large doses of iron can reduce the uptake of zinc and calcium. For healthy bones, a finely tuned balance of vitamin D, calcium, phosphorus, magnesium, zinc, manganese, fluoride, chloride, copper and boron is required. Vitamin C enhances the absorption of iron, converting it from its inactive ferric form to the active ferrous form. Most of the B vitamins are involved in energy metabolism, so a short term shortage of one may be compensated for by a plentiful supply of another.

If in doubt about supplements, it is safest to choose a multi-vitamin and mineral formulation rather than individual supplements. Single supplements should only be considered with the advice of your doctor or nutritionist.

Are natural vitamins better than synthetic?

It has been claimed that 'natural' or 'food source' vitamins are better absorbed than 'synthetic' but, for the majority, there is no proven difference. Most have an identical chemical structure. One exception is vitamin E which is better absorbed in its natural form (d-alpha tocopherol).

Are time release supplements better?

Time release vitamins are coated with protein and embedded in micropellets within the pill. In theory, the supplement should take longer to dissolve, with the protein coating slowing down vitamin absorption. However, there is little evidence that this is the case or that they are better for you. If you take any supplement with a meal, the absorption of the vitamins and minerals is retarded anyway by the carbohydrate/fat/protein in the food. So, it is not worth paying extra money for time release supplements.

How should I choose a supplement?

Here are some basic guidelines.

◆ If in doubt, choose a multivitamin/mineral supplement, ideally one which highlights its antioxidant content.
◆ Check it contains a wide range of vitamins and minerals (vitamins A, C, D, E, beta-carotene, thiamin, riboflavin, niacin, pyridoxine, vitamin B12, folic acid, pantothenic acid, biotin, calcium, iron, zinc).
◆ The amounts of each nutrient should be no more than between 100 and 200% of the RDA stated on the label and, ideally, in the same proportions.

◆ Avoid high dose supplements (i.e. more than 10 times the RDA) – they won't improve health or performance, so are an unnecessary expense.

◆ Expensive brands are not necessarily better for you.

What are free radicals?

Free radicals are atoms or molecules with an unpaired electron and are produced all the time in our bodies as a result of normal metabolism and energy production. They can easily generate other free radicals by snatching an electron from any nearby molecule, and exposure to cigarette smoke, pollution, exhaust fumes, UV light and stress can increase their formation.

In large numbers, free radicals have the potential to wreak havoc in the body. Free radical damage is thought to be responsible for heart disease, many cancers, ageing and post exercise muscle soreness, as unchecked, free radicals can damage cell membranes and genetic material (DNA), destroy enzymes, disrupt red blood cell membranes, and oxidise LDL cholesterol in the bloodstream, thus also increasing the risk of atherosclerosis or the furring of arteries – the first stage of heart disease. Recent studies have demonstrated increased levels of free radicals following exercise and these have been held responsible for muscle soreness, pain, discomfort, oedema (fluid retention) and tenderness post exercise.

The good side of free radicals

Not all free radicals are damaging. Some help to kill germs, fight bacteria and heal cuts. The problem arises when too many are formed and cannot be controlled by the body's defence system.

How can free radicals be controlled?

Fortunately, your body has a number of natural defences against free radicals. They are called antioxidants and work as free radical scavengers, donating one of their own electrons to 'neutralise' the free radicals. They include various enzymes (e.g. superoxide dismutase, glutathione, peroxidase) which have minerals such as manganese, selenium and zinc incorporated in their structure; beta-carotene; vitamins C and E, as well as hundreds of other natural substances in plants, called phytonutrients. These include plant pigments, bioflavanoids, tannins and carotenoids.

Do athletes need more antioxidants?

There is mounting evidence that free radical production is increased by intense exercise and that a plentiful supply of antioxidants can help protect muscle fibres from the resulting damage. A number of studies have shown that athletes given antioxidant supplements experienced less muscle cell damage after strenuous exercise compared with those given a placebo (*see* box page 76). Boosting your antioxidant intake is therefore likely to be beneficial.

A vitamin C supplement may be useful if you are involved in prolonged high intensity training because it may stabilise cell membranes and protect against viral attack. One study found a reduced incidence of upper respiratory tract infections in ultra marathon runners who took 600 mg vitamin C for 21 days prior to the race. Another study at the University of Cape Town found that vitamin C supplements and combined vitamin C/vitamin E/beta-carotene supplements halved the incidence of post race infections.

Since many exercisers have a low zinc intake due to their low food intake overall, scientists say that increasing zinc from dietary sources (rather than from supplements) may help to restore immune function.

Should I take antioxidant supplements?

There is good evidence that antioxidant nutrients (e.g. beta-carotene, vitamins C and E, selenium, bioflavanoids), found chiefly in fresh fruit and vegetables, may help protect against heart disease, certain cancers and post exercise muscle soreness.

Although most of the studies to date point to a positive role for antioxidant supplements, the case is by no means cut and dry. For example, it seems that the positive effects of antioxidant supplements are confined to high intensity exercise and may not apply to lower intensity exercise.

Scientists do not know what the optimal dose is nor whether there are harmful side effects associated with high dose supplements. One study suggested that mega doses may even exacerbate the free radical damage. Until more definitive studies have been carried out, we still need to exercise a certain amount of caution and certainly to avoid indiscriminate supplementation.

The best advice is to aim to get as many antioxidants as possible from food sources as, unlike pills, fruit and vegetables contain a variety of these. The World Health Organisation advise a minimum of five portions (about 400 g) of fruit and vegetables a day. The average intake in the UK is 250 g, so there is plenty of room for improvement.

Plant foods also appear to have other protective substances not present in supplements. When researchers at Cornell University removed the vitamin C from tomato juice, the juice still had cancer fighting properties. Another US study found that people with the highest fruit and vegetable intake had a lower risk of bowel cancer, although those taking supplements of vitamins C, E and beta-carotene did not gain any protective effect.

Which foods are best?

The best source of antioxidants is the natural one: food! There are hundreds of natural substances in food called phytochemicals. These substances found in plant foods have antioxidant properties which are not present in supplements. Each appears to have a slightly different effect and to protect against different types of cancer and other degenerative diseases. For example, the phytochemicals in soya beans may prevent the development of hormone dependent cancers, such as breast, ovarian and prostate cancer [1]. The phytochemicals in garlic can slow down tumour development. It is therefore wise to obtain as wide a range of phytochemicals from food as possible.

How does red wine affect your health?

Evidence is accumulating that red wine may help protect against free radical damage. A study published in *The Lancet* found that red wine drinkers had the lowest risk of heart disease, probably due to its effect of protecting LDL cholesterol from oxidation. This may explain the 'French Paradox'; why the French have such a low rate of heart disease despite their high fat diets and high smoking rate. Red wine contains bioflavanoids from the red grape skins.

1 *Physician and Sportsmed* (23(6), June 1995)

Antioxidant Supplements and Exercise

A recent study by German researchers [2] looked at the effects of vitamin E on the performance of 30 top racing cyclists. The volunteers were divided into two groups. Half were given 330 mg vitamin E (approximately 60 times the average dietary intake) and half were given a placebo for five months. At the end of this period, the supplemented cyclists had considerably greater levels of vitamin E in their blood. All cyclists were then instructed to cycle until the point of exhaustion on a stationary bike. The resistance was increased every five minutes.

Those who had taken supplements had fewer signs of free radical damage, e.g. less leakage of muscle cell enzymes into the blood. The researchers concluded that vitamin E helped to protect the cells from free radical damage, although it had no immediate effect on performance.

Another study by researchers at the University of Göteborg, Sweden, and at the Polish Academy of Sciences tested the effect of a general antioxidant supplement (a pollen extract) on post exercise muscle soreness [3].

Fifty sedentary volunteers were given either the antioxidant supplement or a placebo for four weeks. They then performed an exercise test which included a combination of stepping and cycling at 60–70% of $VO_{2\ max}$. Those who took the antioxidant supplement had less free radical damage and reported less pain, oedema, discomfort and tension in their muscles after exercise.

Researchers concluded that the antioxidant supplement had a beneficial effect.

2 L. Rokitzki et al., α-*Tocopherol Supplementation in Racing Cyclists During Extreme Endurance Training* (International Journal of Sports Nutrition, 4(3), 253–264, 1994)

3 M. Krotkiewski et al., *Prevention of Muscle Soreness by Pretreatment with Antioxidants* (Scandinavian Journal of Medical Science and Sports, 4, 191–199, 1994)

Table 2: *Good sources of antioxidants*

Vitamins *Vitamin C*	Most fruit and veg, especially blackcurrants, strawberries, oranges, tomatoes, broccoli, green peppers, baked potatoes
Vitamin E	Sunflower/safflower/corn oil, sunflower seeds, sesame seeds, almonds, peanuts, peanut butter, avocado, oily fish, egg yolk
Minerals *Selenium*	Wholegrains, vegetables, meat
Copper	Wholegrains, nuts, liver
Manganese	Wheatgerm, bread, cereals, nuts
Zinc	Bread, wholegrain pasta, grains, nuts, seeds, eggs
Carotenoids *Beta-carotene*	Carrots, red peppers, spinach, spring greens, sweet potatoes, mango, cantaloupe melon, dried apricots
Alpha- and gamma-carotene	Red coloured fruit, red and green coloured vegetables
Canthazanthin and lycopene	Tomatoes, watermelon
Flavanoids *Flavanols and polyphenols*	Fruit, vegetables, tea, coffee, red wine, garlic, onions

Are tea and coffee bad for you?

Another study in *The Lancet* found that men with the highest intake of flavanoids (tea was a major source) had fewer heart attacks. As coffee also contains antioxidants, it seems that this too may be beneficial, in moderation.

What are the dangers of low fat diets?

Many health conscious people are cutting down on their fat intake. However, taking this message to the extreme could be dangerous as it means you could be missing out on vitamin E which is found only in oily foods such as seeds, nuts, vegetable oils and egg yolk. Try to include moderate amounts of these foods in your diet regularly otherwise you could be at greater risk of free radical damage.

How much do you need?

In the UK there are no official recommended intakes for any of the antioxidants except vitamin C (40 mg). Several scientists, including Professor Anthony Diplock from the University of London at Guys Hospital, believe the UK and US suggested amounts are too low and Diplock has proposed the following: for beta-carotene, 15–25 mg per day; for vitamin E, 50–80 mg; and for vitamin C, 100–150 mg, all of which are considerably greater than current average intakes. It would be difficult to obtain these levels of vitamin E and beta-carotene from diet alone, so supplements may be the answer. Others are more cautious in making recommendations and go along with the World Health Organisation's fruit and vegetable recommendation.

Antioxidant Tips

- Eat at least 5 portions of fresh fruit and vegetables a day.
- Include nuts and seeds regularly in your diet.
- Eat more fresh fruit for snacks.
- A daily tipple of red wine (1–2 glasses) may be beneficial.
- Add a side salad to your meals.
- Store vegetable oils in a cool dark place and do not re-use heated oil.

SUMMARY OF KEY POINTS

- Vitamin and mineral requirements depend on age, body size, activity level and individual metabolism.
- Dietary Reference Values should be used as a guide for the general population; they are not targets and do not take account of the needs of athletes.
- Regular and intense exercise increases the requirements for a number of vitamins and minerals. However, there are no official recommendations for athletes.
- Low intakes can adversely affect health and performance. However, high intakes exceeding requirements will not necessarily improve performance.
- A well planned, balanced diet, that meets the individual's energy needs, is also likely to provide sufficient vitamins and minerals. Supplements should not take the place of a balanced diet.
- Supplements containing 100–200% of the RNI may be useful for athletes consuming less than 2000 kcal/day and those with erratic eating habits, food intolerances or on a restrictive diet (e.g. vegan).
- Vitamins A, D and B6 and a number of minerals may be toxic in high doses (more than 10 x RNI). Indiscriminate supplementation may lead to nutritional imbalances and deficiencies.
- Increased free radicals are produced during exercise and may be responsible for post exercise muscle soreness. Excessive amounts may also increase the risk of heart disease, certain cancers and premature ageing.
- Antioxidant nutrients can help prevent free radical damage. Therefore, a high dietary intake of antioxidant rich foods is recommended: aim for at least 5 portions of fruit and vegetables a day, with moderate amounts of vegetable oils, oily fish, nuts and red wine.
- The optimal doses for antioxidant nutrients are unknown and the value of supplements not yet clear.

Vitamin	Function(s)	Where found	RNI µg = microgrammes; mg = milligrammes
A	Essential for normal colour vision and for the cells in the eye that enable us to see in dim light; promotes healthy skin and mucous membranes lining the mouth, nose, digestive system, etc.	Liver, meat, eggs, whole milk, cheese, oily fish, butter and margarine	Men: 700 µg/day Women: 600 µg/day
Beta-carotene	Converted into vitamin A (6µg produces 1 µg vitamin A); a powerful antioxidant and free radical scavenger	Brightly coloured fruit and vegetables (e.g. carrots, spinach, apricots, tomatoes)	No official RNI. 15–25 mg is suggested intake
B_1 (Thiamin)	Forms a co-enzyme essential for the conversion of carbohydrates into energy; used for the normal functioning of nerves, brain and muscles	Wholemeal bread and cereals, liver, kidneys, red meat, pulses (beans, lentils and peas)	Men: 0.4 mg/1000 Calories Women: 0.4 mg/1000 Calories
B_2 (Riboflavin)	Required for the conversion of carbohydrates to energy; promotes healthy skin and eyes and normal nerve functions	Liver, kidneys, red meat, chicken, milk, yoghurt, cheese, eggs	Men: 1.3 mg/day Women: 1.1 mg/day
Niacin	Helps to convert carbohydrates into energy; promotes healthy skin, normal nerve functions and digestion	Liver, kidneys, red meat, chicken, turkey, nuts, milk, yoghurt and cheese, eggs, bread and cereals	Men: 6.6 mg/1000 Calories Women: 6.6 mg/1000 Calories

Claim(s) of supplements	The science	Possible dangers of high doses
Maintains normal vision, healthy skin, hair and mucous membranes; may help to treat skin problems such as acne and boils; may affect protein manufacture	Not involved in energy production; little evidence to suggest it can improve sporting performance	Liver toxicity from taking supplements: symptoms include liver and bone damage; abdominal pain; dry skin; double vision; vomiting; hair loss; headaches. May also cause birth defects. Pregnant women should avoid vitamin A supplements and liver. Never exceed 9000 µg/day (men), 7500 µg/day (women)
Reduces risk of heart disease, cancer and muscle soreness	As an antioxidant, may help prevent certain cancers. Other carotenoids in food may also be important	Orange tinge to the skin – probably harmless and reversible
May optimise energy production and performance; is usually present with a B complex or multivitamin	Involved in energy (ATP) production, so the higher the energy expenditure, the higher the thiamin requirement; increased needs can normally be met in the diet (cereals and other foods high in complex carbohydrates); there is no evidence to suggest that high intakes enhance performance; supplements are probably unnecessary	Cannot be stored – excess is excreted therefore unlikely to be toxic; toxic symptoms (rare) may include insomnia, rapid pulse, weakness and headaches. Avoid taking more than 3 g/day
Sportspeople may need more B_2 because they have higher energy needs – supplements may optimise energy production; usually present within a B complex or multivitamin	Forms part of the enzymes involved in energy production, so exercise may increase the body's requirements; however, these can usually be met by a balanced diet; there is no evidence that supplements improve performance; if you take the contraceptive pill you may need extra B_2	Rarely toxic as it cannot be stored; any excess is excreted in the urine (a bright yellow colour)
Sportspeople need more niacin since it is involved in metabolism; higher doses may help to reduce blood-cholesterol levels	Not enough evidence to prove that high doses can help to improve performance; requirements can be met by a balanced diet	Excess is excreted in the urine; doses of more than 200 mg of nicotinic acid may cause dilation of the blood vessels near the skin's surface (hot flushes)

Vitamin	Function(s)	Where found	RNI
B_6 (Pyridoxine)	Involved in the metabolism of fats, proteins and carbohydrates; promotes normal red blood cell formation; is actively used in many chemical reactions of amino acids and proteins	Liver, nuts, pulses, eggs, bread, cereals, fish, bananas	Men: 1.4 mg/day Women 1.2 mg/day
Pantothenic acid (B vitamin)	Involved in the metabolism of fats, proteins and carbohydrates; promotes healthy skin, hair and normal growth; helps in the manufacture of hormones and antibodies, which fight infection; helps energy release from food	Liver, wholemeal bread, brown rice, nuts, pulses, eggs, vegetables	No RNI in the UK
Folic acid (B vitamin)	Essential in the formation of DNA; necessary for red blood cell manufacture	Liver and offal, green vegetables, yeast extract, wheatgerm, pulses	Men: 200 µg/day Women: 200µg/day
B_{12}	Needed for red blood cell manufacture and to prevent some forms of anaemia; used in fat, protein and carbohydrate metabolism; promotes growth and cell development; needed for normal nerve functions	Meat, fish, offal, milk, cheese, yoghurt; vegan sources (fortified foods) are soya protein and milk, yeast extract, breakfast cereals	Men: 1.5 µg/day Women: 1.5 µg/day
Biotin	Involved in the manufacture of fatty acids and glycogen, and in protein metabolism; needed for normal growth and development	Egg yolk, liver and offal, nuts, wholegrain and oats	No RNI in the UK; 10–200 µg day is thought to be a safe and adequate range

Claim(s) of supplements	The science	Possible dangers of high doses
...ortspeople may need ...gher doses to meet their ...creased energy ...quirements	Requirement is related to protein intake, so sportspeople on high-protein diets may need extra B_6; endurance work may cause greater-than-normal losses; there is no evidence to suggest that high doses improve performance; extra doses may help to alleviate PMS (the premenstrual syndrome)	Excess is excreted in the urine; very high doses (over 2 g/day) may cause numbness and unsteadiness
...nce it is involved in ...rotein, fat and ...rbohydrate metabolism, ...ortspeople may need ...gher doses; usually ...resent in a B complex or ...ultivitamin – for overall ...ell-being	No evidence to suggest that high doses improve performance	Excess is excreted in the urine
...upplements help overall ...ell-being, and also ...revent folic acid deficiency ...nd anaemia; these would, ...a theory, hinder aerobic ...erformance	No studies have been carried out on athletic performance and folic acid	Dangers of toxicity are very small, though high doses may reduce zinc absorption
...nce it is involved in the ...evelopment of red blood ...ells, the implication is that ...$_{12}$ can improve the body's ...xygen carrying capacity ...nd therefore its aerobic ...erformance); athletes have ...een known to use ...njections of vitamin B_{12} ...efore competition in the ...ope that it will improve ...heir endurance; usually ...resent within a B complex ...r multivitamin	Extra vitamin B_{12} has no effect on endurance or strength; there is no benefit to be gained from taking supplements (deficiencies are very rare)	Excess is excreted in the urine
...lthough biotin was once ...nown amongst body ...uilders as the 'dynamite ...itamin', no specific role ...or this vitamin in sporting ...erformance has been ...laimed; it is usually ...resent within a B complex ...r multivitamin	The body can make its own biotin, so supplements are unnecessary	There are no known cases of biotin toxicity

Vitamin	Function(s)	Where found	RNI
C	Growth and repair of body cells; collagen formation (in connective tissue) and tissue repair; promotes healthy blood vessels, gums and teeth; haemoglobin and red blood cell production; manufacture of adrenalin; powerful antioxidant	Fresh fruit (especially citrus), berries and currants, vegetables (especially dark green, leafy vegetables), tomatoes and peppers	Men: 40 mg/day Women: 40 mg/day
D	Controls absorption of calcium from the intestine and helps to regulate calcium metabolism; prevents rickets in children and osteomalacia in adults; helps to regulate bone formation	Sunlight (UV light striking the skin), fish oils and oily fish, eggs, vitamin-D-fortified cereals, margarines and some yoghurts	No RNI in the UK
E	As an antioxidant, it protects tissues against free radical damage; promotes normal growth and development; helps in normal red blood cell formation	Pure vegetable oils, wheatgerm, wholemeal bread and cereals, egg yolk, nuts, sunflower seeds, avocado	No RNI in the UK; suggested intake 50–80 mg/day

Mineral	Function(s)	Where found	RNI
Calcium	Important for bone and teeth structure; helps with blood clotting; acts to transmit nerve impulses; helps with muscle contraction	Milk, cheese, yoghurt, soft bones of small fish, seafood, green leafy vegetables, fortified white flour and bread, pulses	Men: 1,000 mg/day Women: 700 mg/day

Claim(s) of supplements	The science	Possible dangers of high doses
Vitamin C may help to increase oxygen uptake and aerobic energy production; exercise causes an increased loss so extra may be needed; intense exercise tends to cause greater free radical damage, so sportspeople need higher doses	A deficiency reduces physical performance; exercise may increase requirements to approximately 80 mg/day – these can be met by including 5 portions of fresh fruit and vegetables in the diet each day; intakes of 100–150 mg may help prevent heart disease and cancer	Excess is excreted, so toxic symptoms are unlikely; high doses may lead to diarrhoea and increase the risk of kidney stones in people who are prone to them
	Not so far shown to be beneficial to performance	Fat-soluble and can be stored in the body; toxicity is rare but symptoms may include high blood pressure, nausea, an irregular heart beat and thirst
Since it is an antioxidant, it may improve oxygen utilisation in the muscle cells; it may also help to protect the cells from the damaging effects of intense exercise; may help to protect against heart disease and cancer	Supplements may have a beneficial effect on performance at high altitudes, and may help reduce heart disease, cancer risk, and post exercise muscle soreness; requirements are related to intake of polyunsaturated fatty acids	Although it cannot be excreted, toxicity is extremely rare

Claim(s) of supplements	The science	Possible dangers of high doses
May help to prevent calcium deficiency and, in some cases, osteoporosis (brittle bone disease)	There is no evidence that extra calcium prevents osteoporosis; exercise (with adequate calcium intake) prevents bone loss, so supplements would seem to be unnecessary; sportspeople who eat few or no dairy products may find calcium supplements useful for meeting basic dietary requirements; extra calcium may help to reduce the risk of stress fractures in sportswomen with menstrual irregularities	The balance of calcium in the bones and blood is finely controlled by hormones – calcium toxicity is thus virtually unknown

Mineral	Function(s)	Where found	RNI
Sodium	Helps to control body fluid balance; involved in muscle and nerve functions	Table salt, tinned vegetables, fish, meat, ready made sauces and condiments, processed meats, bread, cheese	Men: 1.6 g/day (= 4 g salt) Women: 1.6 g/day (= 4 g salt)
Potassium	Works with sodium to control fluid balance and muscle and nerve functions	Vegetables, fruit and fruit juices, unprocessed cereals	Men: 3.5 g/day Women: 3.5 g/day
Iron	Involved in red blood cell formation and oxygen transport and utilisation	Red meat, liver, offal, fortified breakfast cereals, shellfish, wholegrain bread, pasta and cereals, pulses, green leafy vegetables	Men: 8.7 mg/day Women: 14.8 mg/day
Zinc	A component of many enzymes involved in the metabolism of proteins, carbohydrates and fats; helps to heal wounds; assists the immune system; needed for building cells	Meat, eggs, wholegrain cereals, milk and dairy products	Men: 9.5 mg/day Women: 7 mg/day
Magnesium	Involved in the formation of new cells, in muscle contraction and nerve functions; assists with energy production; helps to regulate calcium metabolism; forms part of the mineral structure of bones	Cereals, vegetables, fruit, potatoes, milk	Men: 300 mg/day Women: 270 mg/day
Phosphorus	Assists in bone and teeth formation; involved in energy metabolism as a component of ATP	Cereals, meat, fish, milk and dairy products, green vegetables	Men: 540 mg/day Women: 540 mg/day

Claim(s) of supplements	The science	Possible dangers of high doses
It has been claimed that extra salt is needed if you sweat a lot or exercise in hot, humid conditions; advocated for treating cramp	Excessive sweating during exercise may cause a marked loss of sodium, but as salt is present in most foods, supplements are usually unnecessary; extra salt is more likely to cause, rather than prevent, cramp – dehydration is normally the cause of cramp (together possibly with a shortage of potassium)	High salt intakes may increase blood pressure, risk of stroke, fluid retention and upset the electrolyte balance of the body
May help to reduce blood pressure and encourage sodium excretion	Extra potassium is not known to enhance performance; may help to prevent cramp	Excess is excreted, therefore toxicity is very rare
Extra iron can improve the oxygen-carrying capacity of red blood cells, and therefore improve aerobic performance; can prevent or treat anaemia	Iron-deficiency anaemia can impair performance, especially in aerobic activity; exercise destroys red blood cells and haemoglobin and increases loss of iron, therefore iron requirements of sportspeople may be slightly higher than that of sedentary people; iron is lost through menstruation, so supplements may be sensible for sportswomen	High doses may cause constipation and stomach discomfort; they may also interact with zinc, reducing its absorption
Suggest a possible role in high-intensity and strength exercises; may help to boost the immune system	Studies have failed to show that extra zinc is of any benefit to performance; sportspeople with a zinc deficiency may have an impaired immune system, so an adequate intake is important	High doses may cause nausea and vomiting; they also interfere with the absorption of iron and other minerals
Magnesium status may be related to aerobic capacity	Studies have failed to show that magnesium supplements are beneficial to performance	No evidence that high intakes are harmful
It has been claimed that phosphate loading en-hances aerobic performance and delays fatigue	The consensus is that phosphate loading is of little benefit to performance	High intakes over a long period of time may lower blood calcium levels

Other pills and potions

Sportspeople are always searching for a magic food or nutrient that will improve performance and give them a competitive edge. All athletes, whether top level competitors or fitness participants, want to achieve their best. Being able to achieve that little bit extra by taking a pill or a potion is naturally attractive.

Not surprisingly, then, there is a huge variety of products on the market claiming to help sports performance in some way. These are sometimes called 'ergogenic aids', meaning substances which 'increase work' or 'enhance performance'.

All kinds of images are used by supplement manufacturers. Often these are implied on product labels or advertisements, perhaps by using sporting images and pictures. Scientific claims are frequently exaggerated, with only flimsy evidence or anecdotes to back them up. For example, advertisers may mention a successful 'study' involving a supplement, but they often do not provide details about how many people were involved, how the study was organised and controlled, and how results were treated. They will only tell you about the good findings, not the bad ones.

The 'copy cat' syndrome is common among sportspeople. If someone in your team or club takes a particular supplement and knocks a second off their time, it is tempting to attribute the improved performance to the supplement and therefore to want to try it too. You may have heard about a popular athlete who has tried a product, so you assume that it will make you as good as him. This is why advertisers often use well known sports personalities to endorse their products. The implication is that this product was responsible for the person's success, so if you take it it will do the same for you! The point is that there is no proof that this is the case.

Pills and potions can also be very fashionable. As new types of supplements or packaging designs emerge, they can become quite a sought after 'accessory'. Just as new styles of sports clothing and equipment become trendy, so, too, do nutritional products. Do they work; and are they safe?

This chapter examines some of the most popular pills and potions currently being marketed for sportspeople. It looks at what they contain and examines the claims made for them. Are they backed by scientific research? This chapter considers the evidence and whether they are worth taking. Do they have a physiological benefit, or is it all in the mind? Can they really help someone to achieve that competitive edge?

SUMMARY OF KEY POINTS

- There is little scientific evidence to support supplements' claims to enhance muscle size, mass or strength. Most rely on un-published or unreliable ('pseudo-scientific') evidence, animal studies or purely anecdotal information.
- Products claiming to promote weight loss or enhance fat loss have no scientific basis and do not have any effect on fat oxidation at all.
- Carbohydrate supplements based on glucose polymers can help postpone fatigue, improve endurance and performance during prolonged high intensity exercise.
- There is no scientific evidence to support 'health' products such as ginseng, royal jelly, etc.
- There is equivocal evidence for bicarbonate loading improving performance in high intensity (anaerobic) activities, but it does have a number of major side effects.
- High doses of caffeine can enhance fat oxidation, reduce glycogen depletion and improve endurance during prolonged intense aerobic activities, but it is a diuretic (therefore exacerbating dehydration) and a banned substance above a certain dosage.
- Creatine supplements in doses of 20 g/day for 5 days can in-crease muscle PC levels and help maintain maximum power output longer in high intensity activities such as sprinting. However, their value has not yet been proven for all types of high intensity activities or for non élite athletes.

Supplements	What are they?	The claim(s)	The science
Amino acids	Various combinations are available. 'Free form' amino acids are individual ones mixed together, whereas 'peptides' are short chains, usually derived from the partial breakdown of proteins. 'Full spectrum' amino acids contain all 20, including the eight essential ones. 'Branched chain' formulations consist of leucine, valine and isoleucine in a branched chain configuration, while 'time release' formulations are a mixture of free forms and peptides. Some formulations have added B vitamins, and other nutritional substances such as inosine and oryzanol	Encourage muscle growth and prevent muscle breakdown. Growth hormone (GH) 'promoters' claim to stimulate GH production and increase muscle mass	There is no evidence to suggest that amino acid supplements can increase muscle growth, speed recovery or increase GH production. Relatively large amounts would have to be taken to make a significant difference to total daily intake – possibly in excess of 20 capsules a day – which makes it an expensive supplement.
Bicarbonate	Sodium bicarbonate taken just before anaerobic exercise, e.g. sprinting	Delays fatigue and improves performance during high-intensity, short-term exercise such as sprinting	May help to counteract lactic acid build-up and therefore postpone fatigue. More work needs to be done before recommendations can be made. Side-effects include diarrhoea and stomach ache
Caffeine	A stimulant found in coffee, tea, coca-cola, cocoa and some sports drinks	Increases endurance and reduces fatigue	High doses will increase fat mobilisation and utilisation during aerobic exercise, therefore 'sparing' glycogen. Banned over a certain level by the IOC. A powerful diuretic which may lead to dehydration, and can cause

Carbohydrate/glucose polymer supplements	Come as powders to be mixed with water, or as ready-made liquid drinks. Consist mainly of glucose polymers (maltodextrins), some with added vitamins, minerals or electrolytes, and other nutritional substances	Boost energy, replenish carbohydrate stores after exercise and increase endurance	Provide carbohydrate and fluid in a form that can be rapidly absorbed. Useful for strenuous exercise lasting > 1 hour; for carbohydrate loading; for replenishing glycogen after prolonged exercise; or for athletes with very high carbohydrate needs that cannot be met by food. Will not automatically increase vitality. Include calorie content in your overall daily intake
Carnitine	An amino acid made in the liver, involved in fat transport across mitochondria membrane	Increase fat breakdown during exercise, spare glycogen and increase endurance	There is no scientific evidence to suggest that supplements improve fatty acid transportation, help fat loss or increase endurance
Chromium	Usually sold as chromium picolinate. Good dietary sources include wholegrains, nuts, mushrooms, beans, prunes and seafood	Builds muscle, reduces fat, lowers blood cholesterol and increases stamina	A component of GTF (glucose tolerant factor) required for insulin action. Insulin is an anabolic hormone involved in protein, carbohydrate and fat metabolism; it promotes the uptake of protein and carbohydrate into muscle cells and prevents protein breakdown. There is little scientific support of the claims made for chromium

Supplements	What are they?	The claim(s)	The science
Creatine	Forms phosphocreatine (PC), a high energy compound used to regenerate ATP quickly during maximal bursts of high intensity exercise	Increases performance in anaerobic events; maintains maximal power output for longer	Studies have shown that taking 20 g (4×5 g)/day boosts muscle PC levels, buffers acidity, helps sustain power output for longer and leads to improvements in performance of up to 5%. May be useful for élite power/ strength athletes involved in short sprint-based/power activities, but some studies have failed to show positive effects for non-élite athletes or those involved in endurance activities. The optimal dose and long term effects have not been ascertained. Expensive
Dessicated liver	A concentrated form of dried liver, available in tablet or powder form	Increases stamina	Liver is rich in protein, iron and B_{12}, but there is no proof that supplements increase stamina. It should not be taken by pregnant women
Dibencozide	The co-enzyme of vitamin B_{12} – the physiologically active form of this vitamin	Enhances muscle growth, strength and recovery, and provides an alternative to steroids	One study found dibencozide useful for growth retarded children deficient in B_{12}. No proof in adults and athletes

Fat burners	A combination of choline and inositol, sometimes with lecithin, vitamin B_6, carnitine and methionine	Encourage fat breakdown	Although they are involved in fat metabolism, there is no evidence that taking extra amounts will speed the process up. Lecithin is an emulsifier (and a type of fat itself), and may help reduce high blood cholesterol levels
Frac/ferulic acid/gamma oryzanol	Found in many plants, and is bound to other molecules such as sterols (natural steroid alcohols). Gamma oryzanol consists of ferulic acid bound to a sterol. Frac comes from rice bran, and contains ferulic acid plus free sterols	May increase muscle mass and strength, reduce fat and improve recovery	Poor evidence. Tests suggesting these functions can be criticised on the grounds of small subject numbers and inadequate controls
Ginseng	Comes from the root of a plant grown in Asia and North America. Sold in capsules and powders, as tea and even as a whole root; contains peptides and unidentified substances thought to be a stimulant	Improves stamina and immunity. Also said to increase lifespan	Evidence of beneficial effects is patchy. Different preparations contain different types and amounts of ginsenosides, so effects cannot be predicted. The IOC Committee advise competitors to avoid ginseng, as some preparations may contain banned substances. High doses can cause high blood pressure, sleeplessness and anxiety
Glandulars	Concentrated forms of various animal glands, including adrenals, thymus and spleen	Build muscle and increase the sex drive	No benefits have ever been scientifically proven. Extracts may also contain unwanted antibiotics and pesticides!

Supplements	What are they?	The claim(s)	The science
Inositol	Occurs naturally in many foods. There is no dietary requirement	Promotes energy release, helping you to train harder and for longer	Although it is involved in energy metabolism, there is no proof that it increases energy production
Meal replacement products	Drinks consist of milk protein, sugars (carbohydrate), vitamins, minerals and sometimes added fibre. May also contain 'fat burners' and free form amino acids. Bars and biscuits contain cereals, dried fruit, sugar and fibre	Help to control weight and body fat by replacing one or two meals a day	Convenient, expensive and gimmicky, but not intrinsically slimming! Bars/biscuits high in fat. Do not re-educate eating habits. May perpetuate a sweet tooth and snack habit
Medium chain triglycerides (MCTs)	Fats with a shorter fatty-acid chain than most others – between 8 and 14 carbon atoms	Boost energy, help to reduce fat, and maintain muscle, and provide a readily available energy source. Usually aimed at those dieting for competition	Claims based on studies with rats! Like other fats, MCTs provide 9 kcal. Although they are metabolised via a different route, they may still be converted into body fat
Protein powders	Based on milk proteins (casein, lactalbumen, whey) or milk and egg protein. May also contain amino acids, vitamins, and other nutritional substances that claim to enhance muscle growth. Most are designed to be mixed with milk or fruit juice and come in a variety of flavours	Help to meet your protein needs, and encourage muscle growth	High in protein, providing about 25–30 g of protein per serving. Although training increases protein requirements, it is possible to meet these needs from ordinary foods. There is nothing in the products that enhances muscle growth

	What it is	Claims	Evaluation
Royal jelly	A yellow-white substance produced by worker bees and fed to the queen. 60–70% water, with small amounts of protein, carbohydrate, fat, vitamins and minerals	Increases strength and vitality, reduces fatigue and improves general well-being. Fights colds and other infections and slows ageing	Any reported benefits are likely to be due to a placebo effect. There are more nutrients in a bowl of cornflakes than in a generous dose of royal jelly. Expensive
Smilax officianalis	A sterol found in plants	Stimulates testosterone production and therefore increases muscle growth. Strongly marketed as 'the alternative to steroids'	The claims are not supported by any scientific evidence, and it is doubtful whether sterols are even absorbed by the body to an appreciable extent
Spirulina	A microscopic, blue-green alga that grows wild in brackish lakes in the tropics	Increases energy levels, provides protein and other nutrients, and helps to build red blood cells	There is no evidence that it improves athletic performance. Expensive
Steroid Replacers/Mimics	Combinations of amino acids, vitamins, plant or herb extracts	Produce similar results to anabolic steroids, increasing strength and muscle mass, but without harmful side effects	Supplements come with a strength training and nutrition programme. No evidence that they have any effect on performance, body composition or give similar results to steroids. Any benefits are more likely to be due to the intensive strength training programme and improved diet. Expensive
Superoxide dismutase (SOD)	An enzyme found naturally in body cells. It protects them against oxidation and free radical damage	Slows ageing, helps prevent arthritis and cancer, and aids weight loss	There is no evidence that extra is needed by the body. It is unlikely to survive in the digestive tract, as it is digested by other enzymes

Supplements	What are they?	The claim(s)	The science
Weight gain products	Blends of milk or milk and egg protein and sugars/ maltodextrins. May contain vitamins, minerals, amino acids and various 'ergogenic' substances. Most come in powdered form and are mixed with milk or water	Help you to gain weight. Manufacturers recommend 3–4 servings a day as a supplement to normal meals	Provide a low-bulk form of protein and carbohydrate, giving an extra 400–500 Calories/serving or 1200–2000 extra Calories/day. Help people who find it hard to eat sufficient quantities of food to meet their total daily protein and Calorie requirements. However, the only way to gain muscle mass is through heavy resistance work together with an adequate intake of nutrients

6

Drink and be merry!

Exercise is thirsty work.

Whenever you exercise you lose fluid, not only through sweating but also as water vapour in the air that you breathe out. The harder and longer you exercise, and the hotter and more humid the environment, the more fluid you will lose.

Your body's fluid losses can be very high and, if the fluid is not replaced quickly, dehydration will follow. This will have an adverse effect on your physical performance and health. Exercise will be much harder and you will suffer fatigue sooner.

This chapter explains why it is important to drink fluids to avoid dehydration, when is the best time to drink, and how much to drink. It deals with the timing of fluid intake: before, during and after exercise, and considers the science behind the formulation of sports drinks. Do they offer an advantage over plain water; and can they improve performance? Finally, this chapter looks at the effects of alcohol on performance and health, and gives a practical, sensible guide to drinking.

Why do I sweat?

First, let us consider what happens to your body when you exercise.

When your muscles start exercising, they produce extra heat. In fact, about 75% of the energy you put into exercise is converted into heat, and is then lost. This is why exercise makes you feel warmer. Extra heat has to be dissipated to keep your inner body temperature within safe limits – around 37–38°C. If your temperature rises too high, normal body functions are upset and eventually heat stroke can result.

The major method of heat dispersal during exercise is sweating. Water from your body is carried to your skin via your blood capillaries and as it evaporates you lose heat. For every litre of sweat that evaporates you will lose around 600 Calories (2,500 kJ) of heat energy from your body. (You can lose some heat through convection and radiation, but it is not very much compared with sweating.)

Not surprisingly, fluid losses during exercise can be very high. You lose fluid not only in sweat, but also as water vapour as you breathe out.

How much fluid do I lose?

The amount of sweat that you produce and, therefore, the amount of fluid that you lose, depends on:

♦ how hard you are exercising
♦ how long you are exercising for
♦ the temperature and humidity of your surroundings
♦ you as an individual.

The harder and longer you exercise, and the hotter and more humid the environment, the more fluid you will lose. During one hour's exercise an average person could expect to lose around one litre (two pints) of fluid – and even more in hot conditions. During more strenuous exercise in warm or humid conditions (e.g. marathon running) you could be losing as much as two litres (four pints) an hour.

Some people sweat more profusely than others, even when they are doing the same exercise in the same surroundings. This depends partly on body weight and size (a smaller body produces less sweat), your fitness level (the fitter and better acclimatised to warm conditions you are, the more readily you sweat due to better thermoregulation), and individual factors (some people simply sweat more than others!). In general, women tend to produce less sweat than men, due to their smaller body size and their greater economy in fluid loss. The more you sweat, the more care you should take to avoid dehydration.

You can estimate your sweat loss and, therefore, how much fluid you should drink by weighing yourself before and after exercise. Every 1 kg (2.2 lb) decrease in weight should be replaced with 1 litre (1.76 pints) of fluid.

What are the dangers of dehydration?

An excessive loss of fluid (dehydration) impairs performance and has an adverse effect on health. It places extra strain on the heart, lungs and circulatory system, which means the heart has to work harder to pump blood round your body. Exercise becomes much harder as blood volume decreases and body temperature rises.

A loss of just 2% in your weight will affect your ability to exercise, and performance will deteriorate by 10–20% (i.e. your running time would fall by that amount). If you lose 4%, you may experience nausea, vomiting and diarrhoea. At 5% your performance will decrease by 30%, while an 8% drop will cause dizziness, laboured breathing, weakness and confusion. Greater drops have very serious consequences.

Figure 1: Fluid loss reduces exercise capacity

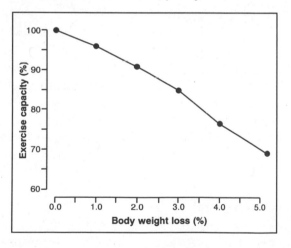

Ironically, the more dehydrated you become, the less able your body is to sweat. This is because dehydration results in a smaller blood volume (due to excessive loss of fluid), and so a compromise has to be made between maintaining the blood flow to muscles and maintaining the blood flow to the surface of the skin to carry away heat. Usually the blood flow to the skin is reduced, causing your body temperature to rise.

If you carry on exercising without replacing fluids you become more and more dehydrated. Your body temperature will increase more and more, and a vicious circle will be set up, resulting eventually in fatigue or heat stroke.

Figure 2: *The dangers of dehydration*

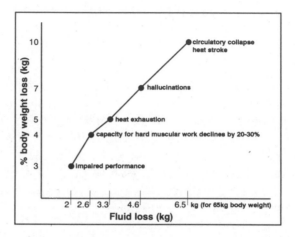

Can I minimise my fluid loss?

You cannot prevent your body from losing fluid. After all, this is a natural and desirable way to regulate body temperature. On the other hand, you can prevent your body from becoming dehydrated by offsetting fluid losses as far as possible. The best way to do this is to make sure you are well hydrated before you start exercising, and to drink plenty of fluids during and after exercise to replace losses.

Are sweat suits a good idea?

Many athletes use sweat suits, plastic, neoprene and other clothing to make weight for competition. This is definitely not a good idea! By preventing sweat evaporation, the clothing prevents heat loss. This will cause your body temperature to rise more and more. In an attempt to expel this excess heat your body will continue to produce more sweat, thus losing increasing amounts of fluid. You will become dehydrated, with the undesirable consequences this entails.

As mentioned above, your ability to exercise will be impaired – you will suffer fatigue much sooner and will have to slow down or stop altogether. Obviously, this is not a good state in which to train or compete.

Losing weight through exercise in sweat suits is not only potentially dangerous, but has no effect whatsoever on fat loss. Any weight loss will simply be fluid, which will immediately be regained when you next eat or drink. The exercise may seem harder because you will be sweating more, but this will not affect the body's rate of fat breakdown. If anything, you are likely to lose less fat, because you cannot exercise as hard or as long when you wear a sweat suit.

When should I drink?

1 Beforehand

Obviously, prevention is better than cure; make sure you are well hydrated *before* you start to exercise by drinking plenty of fluids, especially in hot and humid weather.

If you train in the evening, make sure you have had enough fluids during the day. If you train in the morning, make sure you have plenty to drink first thing before you set out. As a guide, you should be producing a dilute, pale coloured urine. If it looks deep yellow and concentrated, you may be dehydrated and therefore need to drink more.

2 During exercise

As soon as you start exercising, you will start to lose fluid, so try to offset this by drinking at suitable intervals whenever possible. The more you sweat, the more you need to drink. Drink as much as you comfortably can – aim for about a quarter to half a pint every 15 minutes. This may take some getting used to if you do not normally drink anything. If you have found in the past that drinking during exercise makes you feel nauseous, take just the occasional sip to start with. Then get into the habit of taking a few mouthfuls until you become accustomed to taking more fluid. A little is better than none at all.

If you exercise for less than 30 minutes there is less danger of dehydration, and drinking during exercise is probably less important. Make sure, though, that you are well hydrated to start with and that you drink plenty afterwards.

3 Afterwards

Drink freely after exercise to replace your fluid losses. Do not wait until you feel thirsty, as this means you are already dehydrated. Thirst is not a good indicator of body fluid levels.

It is virtually impossible to drink too much – drinking too little is much more often the problem.

Why do I feel nauseous when I drink during exercise?

If you feel nauseous or experience other gastro-intestinal symptoms when you drink, the chances are you are already dehydrated! Even a fairly small degree of dehydration (around 2% of body weight) slows down stomach emptying and upsets the normal rhythmical movement of your gut. This can result in feelings of bloatedness, nausea and vomiting. Avoid this by drinking as much as you comfortably can before exercise and then continue drinking early on in your workout. Do not wait until you feel thirsty or 'save' your drink until the latter stages of your workout!

Is it good to drink water?

Water is a good fluid replacer. This is mostly what you are losing in sweat and what your body needs. For most types of moderate exercise, lasting less than an hour, you cannot go wrong by drinking plenty of water. For longer, more strenuous exercise, you may need the added benefits of another type of drink.

Is it possible to drink too much water?

Drinking too much fluid is very rarely a problem as the body simply excretes any fluid not required. The only circumstance where excessive water may be a problem is during very prolonged or strenuous exercise (e.g. marathon running) when only plain water is drunk and sodium is not replaced. This results in a rapid drop in blood sodium concentration (hyponatraemia) and very watery blood plasma. All this stimulates urine production and reduces the urge to drink, so exacerbating dehydration.

Therefore, if you are sweating heavily for long periods of time, drink dilute electrolyte/carbohydrate drinks rather than plain water. These will help maintain better fluid levels in the body, spare muscle glycogen and thus delay fatigue.

Are sports drinks better?

For many years sports scientists have recommended drinking plain water. In 1984, for example, the American College of Sports Medicine stated that water is the best fluid. However, since then a number of studies have shown that in certain circumstances it may be advantageous to take drinks with added carbohydrate or minerals (electrolytes).

This is because drinking during exercise serves three purposes.

- It can replace water lost through sweating
- It can provide some carbohydrate to spare the body's dwindling reserves of glycogen and maintain blood glucose
- It can provide minerals (electrolytes) to speed water absorption and maintain blood volume.

What are electrolytes?

Electrolytes are mineral salts dissolved in the body's fluid. They include sodium, chloride, potassium and magnesium. They help to regulate the fluid balance between different body compartments: for example, the amount of fluid inside and outside a muscle cell; and the volume of fluid in the circulation. The water movement is controlled by the concentration of electrolytes on either side of the cell membrane. For example, an increase in the concentration of sodium outside a cell will cause water to move to it from inside the cell. Similarly, a drop in sodium concentration will cause water to move from the outside to the inside of the cell.

Can weather affect performance?

Air temperature and wind speed can both affect performance. The hotter and more humid the weather, and the less wind there is, the more fluid your body will lose and the greater the chance of dehydration occurring.

In one study, six athletes cycled on a stationary bike at a set resistance. When the surrounding temperature was 2°C they could cycle for 73 minutes before experiencing exhaustion. When the surrounding temperature increased to 33°C, they could only cycle for 35 minutes. When the athletes were given a carbohydrate drink it was found that they could keep going for longer in cold conditions. However, the drink made no difference in hot conditions.

In hot conditions the body's priority is to replace water rather than carbohydrate. So drink water or a dilute carbohydrate electrolyte drink rather than a more concentrated carbohydrate drink. If you exercise in cold weather and sweat only a little, you may find a more concentrated carbohydrate drink beneficial.

Should I take salt tablets in hot weather?

No, salt tablets are not a good idea, even if you are sweating heavily in hot weather. They produce a very concentrated sodium solution in your stomach (strongly hypertonic), which delays stomach emptying and rehydration as extra fluid must first be absorbed from your body into your stomach to dilute the sodium. The best way to replace fluid and electrolyte losses is by drinking a dilute sodium/carbohydrate drink (either hypotonic or isotonic) with a sodium concentration of 40–110 mg/100 ml.

How can I speed up fluid replacement?

Although plain water is absorbed relatively quickly, the speed can be increased, or decreased, by a number of factors, including:

◆ the volume of fluid drunk
◆ the sugar (carbohydrate) and sodium concentration of the drink
◆ the intensity of exercise.

The larger the volume of fluid in your stomach, the faster it is emptied into the intestines and so the faster it replaces fluid losses in your body. That's why it is best to drink as much as you comfortably can early on in your workout, then to continue topping up with frequent drinks. Obviously, this is easier to do during activities such as cycling, swimming or weight training, where the body is supported or impact is kept to a minimum.

Relatively dilute solutions of sugar and sodium (hypotonic or isotonic) stimulate water absorption from the small intestine into the bloodstream. Sodium actually stimulates both sugar and water absorption, which is why it is added to most commercial sports drinks. A sugar concentration up to approximately 8 g/100 ml and a sodium concentration up to 110 mg/100 ml accelerate water absorption, while more concentrated drinks (hypertonic) slow down the stomach emptying and therefore reduce the speed of fluid replacement. The higher the intensity of exercise, the longer the process takes. Offset this by ensuring you begin your workout well hydrated, and drink a dilute sugar/sodium drink instead of water.

What is the best composition of a sports drink?

There is an optimal concentration range for both sugar and sodium (*see* fig. 3). Studies have shown that a sugar concentration between 4 g and 8 g per 100 ml results in the fastest water absorption. The optimal sodium concentration is between 40 and 110 mg per 100 ml. Although slightly higher sodium concentrations speed water absorption even further, the drink becomes unpalatable. It is important to reach a good compromise between taste and sodium content.

If your fluid losses are very small (e.g. during cool conditions) and you are exercising hard, a more concentrated carbohydrate/energy drink, containing up to 15 g per 100 ml, may be more beneficial in sparing muscle glycogen and delaying fatigue.

What types of sports drinks are available?

Sports drinks can be divided into two main categories: fluid replacement drinks and carbohydrate (energy) drinks.

- **Fluid replacement drinks** are dilute solutions of electrolytes (although the only one worth including is sodium) and sugars (carbohydrate). The sugars most commonly added are glucose,

Figure 3: *Designing the perfect sports drink. Maximal fluid and carbohydrate absorption = 3 g–8 g carb/100 ml*

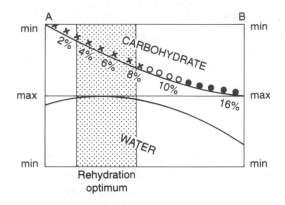

sucrose, fructose and glucose polymers (maltodextrins). The main aim of these drinks is to replace fluid faster than plain water, although the extra sugars will also help maintain blood sugar levels and spare glycogen.

◆ **Carbohydrate (energy) drinks** provide more carbohydrate per 100 ml than fluid replacement drinks. The carbohydrate is mainly in the form of glucose polymers (maltodextrins). The main aim is to provide larger amounts of carbohydrate but at a lower or equal osmolality than the same concentration of glucose. They will, of course, provide fluid as well.

What does osmolality mean?

Osmolality is a measure of the number of dissolved particles in a fluid. A drink with a high osmolality means that it contains more particles per 100 ml than one with a low osmolality. These particles may include sugars, sodium or other electrolytes. The osmolality of the drink determines which way the fluid will move across a membrane (e.g. the gut wall). For example, if a drink with a relatively high osmolality is consumed, then water moves from the bloodstream and gut cells into the gut. This is called *net secretion*. If a drink with a relatively low osmolality is consumed, then water is absorbed from the gut (i.e. the drink) to the gut cells and bloodstream. Thus there is *net water absorption*.

What is the difference between hypotonic, isotonic and hypertonic drinks?

♦ **A hypotonic drink** has a relatively low osmolality, which means it contains fewer particles (sugars and electrolytes) per 100 ml than the body's own fluids. As it is more dilute, it is absorbed faster than plain water. Typically, a hypotonic drink contains less than 4 g sugar/100 ml.

♦ **An isotonic drink** has the same osmolality as the body's fluids, which means it contains about the same number of particles (sugars and electrolytes) per 100 ml and is therefore absorbed as fast as or faster than plain water. Most commercial isotonic drinks contain between 4 and 8 g sugar per 100 ml. In theory, isotonic drinks provide the ideal compromise between rehydration and refuelling.

♦ **A hypertonic drink** has a higher osmolality than body fluids, as it contains more particles (sugars and electrolytes) per 100 ml than the body's fluids, i.e. it is more concentrated. This means it is absorbed more slowly than plain water. A hypertonic drink usually contains more than 8 g sugars per 100 ml.

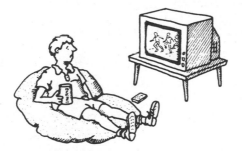

What are glucose polymers?

Between a sugar (1–2 units) and a starch (several 100,000 units), although closer to the former, are glucose polymers (maltodextrins). These are chains of between 4 and 20 glucose molecules produced from boiling cornstarch under controlled commercial conditions.

The advantage of using glucose polymers instead of glucose or sucrose in a drink is that a higher concentration of carbohydrate can be achieved (usually between 10 and 20 g/100 ml) at a lower osmolality. That's because each molecule contains several glucose units yet still exerts the same osmotic pressure as just one molecule of glucose. So an isotonic or hypotonic drink can be produced with a carbohydrate content greater than 8 g/100 ml.

Also, glucose polymers are less sweet than simple sugars, so you can achieve a fairly concentrated drink that does not taste too sickly. In fact, most glucose polymer drinks are fairly tasteless unless they have added artificial flavours or sweeteners.

Do electrolytes improve performance?

Electrolytes in sports drinks do not have any direct effect on performance. The reason they are added to sports drinks is essentially to speed up water absorption and replace sweat losses. However, sodium is the only electrolyte that stimulates water and sugar absorption, the others (such as potassium or magnesium) having no effect at all.

Although small quantities of electrolytes are lost in sweat, they are easily replaced by food. Even if you sweat profusely, loss of electrolytes poses no problem, since your sweat becomes more dilute the longer and harder you exercise.

Do sports drinks improve performance?

Many studies since the 1970s have shown that sports drinks containing small amounts of sodium and carbohydrate can indeed improve performance. They 'work' by virtue of the fact that they deliver water and fuel to the body fast, thus helping the athlete avoid dehydration and delay glycogen depletion.

Most of the studies suggesting a positive effect have been carried out on trained athletes exercising at moderate to high intensities under fairly severe laboratory conditions. Remember, this may differ from your exercise situation. For example, if you are working out at a lower intensity for an hour or less, then plain water may produce an equal performance to a sports drink at a fraction of the price! On the other hand, sports drinks are unlikely to have an adverse effect on your performance and are advantageous for most activities lasting an hour or more.

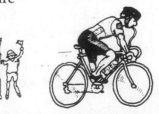

Sports drinks and performance

- In a study carried out at Aberdeen University, cyclists drank either flavoured water or a carbohydrate/electrolyte sports drink, while exercising at 70% VO_{2max} on a stationary bike. The sports drink enabled the cyclists to continue exercising 20 minutes longer than the water.
- In a study at the University of South Carolina, cyclists who consumed a sports drink containing 6 g sugar to 100 ml achieved a faster time trial than those who consumed water.
- In a study at the University of Texas, cyclists who consumed a glucose polymer drink during a time trial were able to continue 31 minutes longer than those drinking plain water.
- At the University of Ohio, recreational cyclists who were given a glucose polymer drink containing 1.1 g or 2.2 g carbohydrate per kg body weight, one hour prior to exercise, completed a laboratory time trial 12.5% faster than those cyclists who drank water.

Which type of drink is best for me?

The type of drink you should choose depends on the intensity and duration of your workout, the temperature and humidity of your surroundings, and how profusely you sweat.

The first factor to consider is whether rapid fluid or fuel replacement is your priority. If you are exercising for less than 60–90 minutes, under very warm and humid conditions and sweating profusely, then rapid fluid replacement is likely to be your priority. Therefore, a fluid replacer (hypotonic or isotonic sports drink) would be best. Choose water if you are exercising at a low or moderate intensity for less than one hour. The choice of a hypotonic or isotonic drink is largely down to personal preference. Although isotonic drinks provide more fuel, some athletes find them a little too concentrated and experience greater fullness or stomach discomfort.

If you are exercising strenuously for more than 90 minutes or under cool conditions and not sweating very much, then fuel replacement is likely to be a greater priority than rapid fluid replacement. Under these circumstances, glycogen depletion is more likely than dehydration to cause early fatigue. Carbohydrate (energy) drinks based on glucose polymers may be a better choice because they can provide more fuel than fluid replacers as well as reasonable amounts of fluid. However, many athletes find that carbohydrate drinks cause stomach discomfort and that fluid replacers containing 4–8 g sugar per 100 ml do an equally good job.

The key is to experiment with different drinks in training to find which one suits you best.

Table 1: *Choosing the right sports drink*

Exercise Conditions	Sports Drink
Exercise lasting < 30 minutes	Nothing, water
Low-moderate intensity exercise lasting < 1 hour	Water, hypotonic or isotonic sports drink
Strenuous exercise lasting 1–2 hours	Hypotonic or isotonic sports drink
Strenuous exercise lasting > 90 min or > 1 hour under cool conditions	Hypotonic or isotonic sports drink, carbohydrate (glucose polymer) drink

What about ordinary soft drinks and fruit juice?

Ordinary soft drinks (typically between 9 and 20 g sugars per 100 ml) and fruit juices (typically between 11 and 13 g sugars per 100 ml) are too concentrated to be used as fluid replacers during exercise. They empty more slowly from the stomach than plain water because they must first be diluted with water from the body, thus causing a net reduction in body fluid. In fact, they can exacerbate dehydration!

If you dilute one part fruit juice with one part water, you will get an isotonic drink, ideal for rehydrating and refuelling during or after exercise (*see* DIY drinks, page 113).

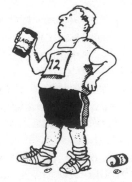

What about diet drinks?

'Diet' or low calorie drinks contain artificial sweeteners in place of sugars and have a very low sodium concentration. They are, therefore, useless as fuel replacers during exercise, although they will help replace fluid at approximately the same speed as plain water. Artificial sweeteners have no known advantage or disadvantage on performance. Choose these types of drink only if you dislike the taste of water, and under the same circumstances that you would normally choose water, i.e. for low to moderate intensity exercise lasting less than 1 hour.

Should I choose still or carbonated drinks?

Experiments at East Carolina University and Ball State University found that carbonated and still sports drinks produced equal hydration in the body. However, the carbonated drinks tended to produce a higher incidence of mild heartburn and stomach discomfort. In practice, many athletes find that carbonated drinks make them feel full and 'gassy', which may well limit the amount they drink. Others actually prefer lightly carbonated to still drinks, so it is really down to individual preference.

Are caffeinated drinks a good idea?

Coffee, tea, cola and a number of new 'sports' drinks contain caffeine (or guarana), a stimulant that has been shown to improve performance in both endurance and sprint based activities. It can also improve alertness and lift your mood. The exact mechanism is not clear, but it is thought that caffeine enhances fatty acid oxidation and spares glycogen utilisation during exercise – effects desired by most athletes.

However, there are a number of disadvantages with caffeinated drinks, which must be taken into account. Firstly, caffeine is a diuretic, causing the body to excrete more water. Secondly, on some people it has the adverse effects of causing anxiety and rapid heart beat. Thirdly, the International Olympic Committee has banned caffeine at levels over 12 μg/1 in the urine (equivalent to drinking 6 cups of instant coffee or 9 cans of cola). The safest advice is to keep off caffeinated drinks before, during or after exercise if you wish to avoid dehydration, are sensitive to its side effects or are competing in a drug-tested competition.

Table 2: *Caffeine content of various drinks*

Drink	mg caffeine per cup
Ground coffee	80–90 mg
Instant coffee	60 mg
Decaffeinated coffee	3 mg
Tea	40 mg
Can of cola	40 mg

Table 3: *Fluid replacement sports drinks*

Hypotonic	Isotonic
◆ Water ◆ 'Diet'/low calorie soft drinks ◆ Diluted squash (1:6) ◆ Diluted fruit juice (1:3) ◆ Dexters ◆ Isostar Light ◆ Lucozade Low Cal Sport ◆ Replay	◆ Diluted squash (1:4) ◆ Diluted fruit juice (1:1) ◆ Isostar ◆ Lucozade Sport ◆ Gatorade ◆ Iso-Buzz ◆ Hydra Fuel

Table 4: *Carbohydrate sports drinks*

◆ Ultra Fuel
◆ Maxim
◆ Long Energy
◆ PSP 22
◆ Top Form
◆ Leppin Carbobooster/Endurobooster
◆ H5 Energy Source
◆ Ultra Carbo
◆ Exceed Carbomax
◆ Carbo Force

Can I make my own sports drinks?

Definitely! Commercial sports drinks work out very expensive if you are drinking at least 1 litre per day to replace fluid losses during exercise. (If you need to drink less than 1 litre then you probably don't need a sports drink anyway.)

Below are some recipes for making your own sports drink.

Table 5: *DIY sports drinks*

Hypotonic	Isotonic
◆ 20–40 g sucrose 1 litre warm water 1–1.5 g salt Sugar-free/low calorie squash for flavouring (optional)	◆ 40–80 g sucrose 1 litre warm water 1–1.5 g salt Sugar-free/low calorie squash for flavouring (optional)
◆ 100 ml fruit squash 900 ml water 1–1.5 g salt	◆ 200 ml fruit squash 800 ml water 1–1.5 g salt
◆ 250 ml fruit juice 750 ml water 1–1.5 g salt	◆ 500 ml fruit juice 500 ml water 1–1.5 g salt

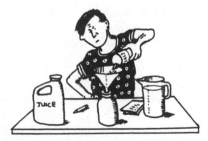

How does alcohol affect my performance?

Drinking alcohol before exercise may appear to make you more alert and confident but, even in small amounts, it will certainly have the following negative effects.

- ◆ Reduce co-ordination, reaction time, balance and judgement.
- ◆ Reduce strength, power, speed and endurance.
- ◆ Reduce your ability to regulate body temperature.
- ◆ Reduce blood sugar levels and increase the risk of hypoglycaemia.

◆ Increase water excretion (urination) and the risk of dehydration.
◆ Increase the risk of accident or injury.

Table 6: *Alcoholic and calorie contents of drinks*

Drink equivalent to 1 unit	% alcohol by volume	Calories
½ pint ordinary beer/lager	3.0–3.5	90
1 measure spirits	38	50
1 measure vermouth/aperitif	18	60–80
4 fl oz glass of wine	11	75–100
1 measure sherry	16	55–70
1 measure liqueur	40	75–100

Can I drink alcohol on non training days?

There is no reason why you cannot enjoy alcohol in moderation on non training days. The Department of Health recommend up to 4 units a day for men and 3 units a day for women as a safe upper limit. The daily limits are intended to discourage binge-drinking which is dangerous to health.

In fact, research has shown that alcohol drunk in moderation reduces the risk of heart disease. Moderate drinkers have a lower risk of death from heart disease than teetotallers or heavy drinkers. The exact mechanism is not certain, but it may work by increasing HDL cholesterol levels, the protective type of cholesterol in the blood. HDL transports cholesterol *back* to the liver for excretion, thereby reducing the chance of it sticking to artery walls. It may also reduce the stickiness of blood platelets, thus reducing the risk of blood clots (thrombosis).

Red wine, in particular, may be especially good for the heart. Studies have shown that drinking up to two glasses a day can lower heart disease risk by 30–70%. It contains flavanoids from the grape skin, which have an antioxidant effect and thus protect the LDL cholesterol from free radical damage.

Is alcohol fattening?

Any food or drink can be 'fattening' if you consume more calories than you need. Alcohol itself provides 7 kcal/g, and many alcoholic drinks also have quite a high sugar/carbohydrate content, boosting the total calorie content further (*see* Table 6). Excess calories from alcoholic drinks can, therefore, lead to fat gain.

What exactly happens to alcohol in the body?

When you drink alcohol, about 20% is absorbed into the bloodstream through the stomach and the remainder through the small intestine. Most of this alcohol is then broken down in the liver (it cannot be stored as it is toxic) into a substance called acetyl CoA and then, ultimately, into ATP (energy). Obviously, whilst this is occurring, less glycogen and fat are used to produce ATP in other parts of the body.

However, the liver can only carry out this job at a fixed rate of approximately 1 unit of alcohol per hour. If you drink more alcohol than this, it is dealt with by a different enzyme system in the liver (the microsomal ethanol oxidising system, MEO) to make it less toxic to the body. The more alcohol you drink on a regular basis, the more MEO enzymes are produced, which is why you can develop an increased tolerance to alcohol – you need to drink more to experience the same physiological effects.

Initially, alcohol reduces inhibitions, increases self confidence and makes you feel more at ease. However, it is actually a depressant rather than a stimulant, reducing your psychomotor (co-ordination) skills. It is potentially toxic to all of the cells and organs in your body and, if it builds up to high concentrations, can cause damage to the liver, stomach and brain.

Too much alcohol causes hangovers – headache, thirst, nausea, vomiting and heartburn. These symptoms are due partly to dehydration and a swelling of the blood vessels in the head. Congeners, substances found mainly in darker alcoholic drinks such as rum and red wine, are also responsible for many of the hangover symptoms. Prevention is better than cure, so make sure you follow the guidelines on page 116. The best way to deal with a hangover is to drink plenty of water or, better still, a sports drink. Avoid coffee or tea as these will make dehydration worse. Do not attempt to train or compete with a hangover!

Sensible drinking guidelines

- Intersperse alcoholic drinks with water, diluted juice or other non alcoholic drinks.
- Extend your alcoholic drink (e.g. wine, spirits) with water, low calorie mixers or soda water.
- Keep a tally on your alcohol intake when you go out; set yourself a safe limit.
- If you think you have drunk too much, drink plenty of water/sports drink before retiring to bed – at least 1 pint per 2–3 units.
- Do not feel obliged to drink excessively, even if your friends press you: tell them you are training the next day or that you are driving.
- Do not drink on an empty stomach as this speeds alcohol absorption. Try to eat something first or reserve drinking for mealtimes. Food slows down the absorption of alcohol.

SUMMARY OF KEY POINTS

- Dehydration impairs performance and health.
- Fluid losses during exercise depend on exercise duration and intensity; temperature and humidity; body size; fitness level and the individual. They can be as high as 1–2 l/hour.
- Always start exercise well hydrated. Continue drinking at regular intervals early on and drink plenty afterwards to fully replace fluid losses.
- Water is a suitable fluid replacement drink for moderate exercise, lasting less than 1 hour.
- For more intense exercise, lasting more than 1 hour, dilute solutions of sodium and carbohydrate can speed up water absorption and provide additional fuel.
- The optimal concentration for a fluid replacement sports drink is 4–8 g carbohydrate per 100 ml and 40–110 mg sodium per 100 ml. However, a compromise between function and taste is often made in commercial drinks.

- Hypotonic (< 4%) and isotonic (4–8%) sports drinks are most suitable when rapid fluid replacement is the main priority.
- Carbohydrate drinks based on glucose polymers also replace fluids, but provide greater amounts of carbohydrate (10–20%) at a lower osmolality. They are most suitable for prolonged intense exercise (> 90 min), when fuel replacement is a major priority or fluid losses are small.
- Alcohol before exercise has a negative effect on strength, endurance, co-ordination, power and speed and increases injury risk.
- Moderate amounts of alcohol (< 4 units/day for men; < 3 units/day for women) in the overall diet, particularly red wine, which is rich in antioxidants, may protect against heart disease.

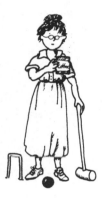

Fat matters

As athletes in almost every sport strive to get leaner and competitive standards get higher, the relationship between body fat, health and performance becomes increasingly important. However, the optimal body composition for fitness or sports performance is not necessarily a desirable one from a health point of view. This chapter deals with the different methods for measuring body fat percentage and body fat distribution, and considers their relevance to performance. It highlights the dangers of attaining very low body fat levels as well as the risks associated with a very low fat diet. It gives realistic guidance on recommended body fat ranges and fat intakes, and explains the difference between the various types of fats found in the diet.

Can excess fat affect performance?

Carrying around excess body weight in the form of fat is a distinct disadvantage in almost every sport. It can adversely affect strength, speed and endurance. Surplus fat is basically surplus baggage. Carrying around this extra weight is not only unnecessary, but also costly in terms of energy expenditure.

For example, in endurance sports, such as long distance running, surplus fat can reduce speed and increase fatigue. It is like carrying a couple of shopping bags with you as you run; they make it harder for you to get up speed, slow you down and cause you to tire quickly. It is best to leave your shopping bags at home, or at least to lighten the load.

In explosive sports, such as sprinting and jumping, where you

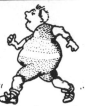

must transfer or lift the weight of your whole body very quickly, extra fat again is non-functional weight, slowing you down, reducing your power and decreasing your mechanical efficiency. Muscle is useful weight, whereas excess fat is not.

In weight matched sports, such as boxing, karate, judo and lightweight rowing, greater emphasis is put on body weight, particularly during the competitive season. The person with the greatest percentage of muscle and the smallest percentage of fat has the advantage.

In fact, in all sports where you must support your body weight – football, squash, skating and tennis, to name but a few – fatness is a disadvantage. The fatter athletes tend to be slower than the lean athletes in these sports, and they tire more easily.

Is fat an advantage in certain sports?

Until recently, it was believed that extra weight – even in the form of fat – was an advantage for certain sports in which momentum is important, such as discus and hammer throwing, judo and wrestling.

A heavy body can generate more momentum to throw an object or knock over an opponent, but there is no reason why this weight should be fat. It would be better if it were in the form of muscle. Muscle is stronger and more powerful than fat – although, admittedly, it is harder to acquire! If two athletes both weighed 100 kg, but one comprised 90 kg lean (10 kg fat) mass, and other 70 kg lean (30 kg fat) mass, the leaner one would obviously have the advantage. Perhaps the only sport where fat could be considered a necessary advantage is sumo wrestling – it would be almost impossible to acquire a very large body mass without fat gain.

What does body composition mean?

The body is composed of two elements: lean body tissue (i.e. muscles, organs, bones and blood) and body fat or adipose tissue. The proportion of these two components in the body is called body composition. This is more important than total weight.

For example, two people may weigh the same, but have a different body composition. Athletes usually have a smaller percentage of body fat and a higher percentage of lean weight than less physically active people. Lean body tissue is functional (or useful) weight, whereas fat is non-functional in terms of sports performance.

How can I tell if I am too fat?

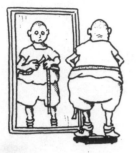

Looking in the mirror is the quickest and simplest way to see if you are too fat by everyday standards, but will not give the accurate information that you need for your sport. Many women also tend to perceive themselves as fatter than they really are. It is useful therefore to employ some sort of measurement system so that you can work towards a definite goal.

Standing on a set of scales, reading your weight and comparing it to standard weight and height charts is easy. However, it has several drawbacks. Weights and heights given in charts are based on average weights of a sample population. They are only *average* weights for *average* people, not ideal weights, and give no indication of health risk.

What is the Body Mass Index?

Doctors and researchers often use a measurement called the Body Mass Index (BMI) to classify different grades of body weight and to assess health risk. It is sometimes referred to as the Quetelet Index after the Belgian researcher who observed that, for normal weight people, there is more or less a constant ratio between weight and the square of height. The BMI assumes that there is no single ideal weight for a person of a certain height, and that there is a healthy weight range for any given height.

The BMI is calculated by dividing a person's weight (in kg) by the square of his or her height (in m). For example, if your weight is 60 kg and height 1.7 m, your BMI is 21.

$$\frac{60}{1.7 \times 1.7} = 21$$

Table 1: *BMI classification*

< 20	Underweight	↑ increasing health risk
20–24.9	'Normal' weight (Grade 0)	lowest health risk
25–29.9	Overweight/'plump' (Grade I)	
30–40	Moderately obese (Grade II)	increasing health risk
40+	Severely obese (Grade III)	↓

Overweight statistics in England

The 1993 OPCS Health Survey found that, in England, 57% of men and 48% of women are overweight (BMI > 25), with a higher incidence of obesity (BMI > 30) occurring in women.

Table 2: *Overweight statistics in England*

	O/weight	Obese	Total
Men	44%	13%	57%
Women	32%	16%	48%

The BMI has a number of limitations. It does not give information about body composition, i.e. how much weight is fat and how much lean tissue. It simply gives the desirable weight of *average* people – not *sportspeople*!

When you stand on the scales you weigh everything – bone, muscle and water, as well as fat. Therefore you do not know how fat you actually are. Someone with a lot of muscle but little fat could be classed as overweight, and vice versa – someone with a relatively high proportion of fat and little muscle could be classed as of average weight.

How useful is the BMI?

Researchers and doctors use BMI measurements to assess a person's risk of acquiring certain health related conditions, such as heart disease. Studies have shown that people with a BMI of between 20 and 25 have the lowest risk of developing diseases that are linked to obesity, e.g. cardio-vascular disease, gall bladder disease, hypertension (high blood pressure) and diabetes. People with a BMI of between 25 and 30 are at moderate risk, while those with a BMI above 30 are at a greater risk.

It is not true that the lower a person's BMI the better, though. A very low BMI is also not desirable; people with a BMI below 20 have a higher risk of other health problems, such as respiratory disease, certain cancers and metabolic complications.

Both those with a BMI below 20 and those above 30 have an increased risk of premature death (*see* fig. 1).

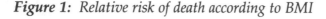

Figure 1: *Relative risk of death according to BMI*

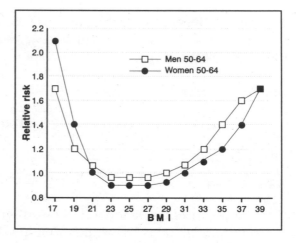

Is the distribution of body fat important?

Yes. Scientists believe that the distribution of your body fat is more important than the total amount of fat. This gives a more accurate assessment of your risk of metabolic disorders, such as heart disease, maturity onset diabetes, high blood pressure and gall bladder disease. Fat stored mostly around the abdomen (central or android obesity) gives rise to an 'apple' or 'barrel' shape, and this carries a much bigger health risk than fat stored mostly around the hips and thighs (peripheral or gynecoid obesity) in a pear shape.

The way we distribute fat on our body is determined partly by our genetic make up and partly by our natural hormonal balance. Men, for example, have higher levels of testosterone, which favours fat deposition around the abdomen, between the shoulder blades and close to the internal organs. Women have higher levels of oestrogen, which favours fat deposition around the hips, thighs, breasts and triceps. After the menopause, however, when oestrogen levels fall, fat tends to transfer from the hips and thighs to the abdomen, giving women more of an apple shape and pushing up their chances of heart disease.

How can I measure my body fat distribution?

You can assess your body fat distribution by the *Waist: Hip Ratio*, which is simply your waist measurement (in inches or centimetres) divided by your hip measurement. For women, (because of their proportionately larger pelvic hip bones) it should be on or below 0.8. For men, this ratio should be less than 0.95. For example, a woman with a waist measurement of 26" (66 cm) and hips of 36" (91.4 cm), has a W/H ratio of 0.72 (26 ÷ 36).

A value greater than the recommended threshold indicates excess fat in the abdomen and a higher health risk. For example, a man with a W/H ratio of 1.1 has double the chance of having a heart attack than if it was below 0.95. The most likely explanation is to do with the close proximity of the intra-abdominal fat to the liver. Fatty acids from the adipose tissue are delivered into the portal vein that goes directly to the liver. The liver thus receives a continuous supply of fat-rich blood and this stimulates increased cholesterol synthesis. High blood cholesterol levels are a major risk factor for heart disease.

How can I measure my body fat?

There are a number of methods for working out the percentage of body fat.

1 Skinfold measurement

Skinfold thickness is measured at various points on the body by a trained person using special calipers. The four most commonly used points are the back of the upper arm (triceps), the top of the upper arm (biceps), beneath the shoulder blade (subscapular), and just above the hip bone (supriliac). The sum of these measurements is read off on an equation chart, which then gives a body fat percentage. The calculations assume that the amount of fat under the skin is proportional to the total amount of fat in the body. Allowances are made for age and sex in the equations.

Many health clubs and sports centres use this method, as it is quick, relatively simple to carry out, and cheap. However, it has a number of drawbacks. It relies heavily on the accuracy of the person taking the measurements. Also, it assumes that everyone of a certain age and sex has a similar pattern of fat distribution. It is not very accurate for athletes, as they tend to have a different pattern of fat distribution from non active people. It is not an accurate method for very lean or very fat people, either.

Physiologists recommend simply recording skinfold thickness, without converting it into a body fat percentage. Together with simple girth measurements, they are useful for monitoring body composition changes over a period of time.

2 Underwater weighing

A person is weighed when submerged under water, and then again on dry land. The two readings are used to calculate body *density*, the principle being that fat is more buoyant than muscle or bone. The figures are then used to work out the percentage weight of body fat.

This method is often judged to be the most accurate and is used as the standard against which other methods can be compared. However, the equipment is sophisticated, expensive and not widely available in this country.

3 Bio-electrical impedence

An electrode is attached to the foot and hand, and a very mild electrical current passed between them. Body fluids and electrolytes conduct the current. Body fat creates a resistance, so the body fat percentage can be calculated by the amount of electrical resistance met. This is an easy, quick and safe method, requiring little training, and the small units are portable. However, changes in body fluid levels and skin temperature may affect readings, making them somewhat unreliable.

4 Near-infra-red interactance

An infra-red beam is shone perpendicularly through the upper arm. The amount of light reflected back to the analyser from the bone depends on the amount of fat in the arm, which is correlated to body fat percentage. Age, weight, height, sex and activity level are all taken into account in the calculations.

The obvious disadvantage to this method is the assumption that fat in the arm is proportional to total body fat. However, it is a very fast, easy and cheap method. The equipment is portable, and anyone can operate it.

How accurate are these methods?

The underwater weighing method is generally regarded as the most accurate, particularly for athletes. A number of studies carried out at the Dunn Clinical Nutrition Centre in Cambridge and Loughborough University found that skinfold thickness (provided it was measured by a well trained person) was the next most reliable method, followed by electrical impedence and near-infra-red interactance.

Table 3: *Accuracy of body fat measurement methods*

Method	Degree of accuracy
Skinfold measurement	4%
Underwater weighing	3%
Electrical impedence	> 5%
Near-infra-red interactance	5–10%

Should I aim to be fat free?

Definitely not! A fat free body would not survive. It is important to realise that some body fat is absolutely vital. This is called essential fat and includes the fat which forms part of your cell membranes, brain tissue, nerve sheaths, bone marrow and the fat surrounding your organs (e.g. heart, liver, kidneys). Here it provides insulation, protection and cushioning against physical damage. In a healthy person, this accounts for about 3% of body weight.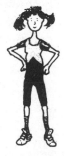

Women have an additional fat requirement called sex specific fat, which is stored mostly in the breast and around the hips. This fat accounts for a further 5–9% of a woman's body weight and is involved in oestrogen production as well as the conversion of inactive oestrogen into its active form. So, this fat ensures normal hormonal balance and menstrual function. If stores fall too low, hormonal imbalance and menstrual irregularities result, although these can be reversed once body fat increases. There is some recent evidence that a certain amount of body fat in men is necessary for normal hormone production too (*see* page 128).

Do I really need fat as an energy reserve?

Fat is also an important energy store, providing 9 kcal/g. It is used virtually all the time during any aerobic activity: while sleeping, sitting, standing and walking, as well as in most types of exercise. This fat comes from adipose tissue distributed all over your body and also from the fat within the muscle cells (this is particularly important during exercise). It is impossible to selectively spot reduce fat from adipose tissue sites by specific exercises or diets. The body generally uses fat from all sites, although the exact pattern of fat utilisation (and storage) is determined by your genetic make up and hormonal balance. An average person has enough fat for three days and three nights of continuous running – although, in practice, you would experience fatigue long before your fat reserves ran out. So, your fat stores are certainly not a redundant depot of unwanted energy!

What is a desirable body fat percentage for health?

Doctors and physiologists recommend a minimum of 5% for men and 10% for women to cover the most basic functions. In practice, a healthy range for men is between 13% and 18% and for women, between 18% and 25%. Sportspeople are likely to be a little lower. Our study of élite athletes found men had 4–10% body fat and women 13–18%. However, these are not necessarily recommended levels for health.

It is important to realise that there is not a straightforward, linear relationship between body fat percentage and performance – everyone has their own individual optimal fat level at which they will perform best. That's why there is no ideal body fat percentage for any particular sport, rather a range of values (*see* Table 4).

Table 4: *Average body fat percentages in various sports*

	Men (%)	Women (%)
Basketball	7–12	18–27
Bodybuilding (competitive)	6–7	8–10
Cycling	8–9	15–16
Football	8–18	
Gymnastics	3–6	8–18
Swimming	4–10	12–23
Running	4–12	8–18
Throwing	12–20	22–30
Tennis	12–16	22–26
Weight lifting	6–16	17–20

What are the dangers for women of attaining very low body fat levels?

One of the biggest problems for women with very low body fat levels is the resulting hormonal imbalance and amenorrhoea (absence of periods). This tends to be triggered once body fat levels fall below 15–20% – the threshold level varies from one person to another. This fall in body fat is sensed by the hypothalamus of the brain, which then decreases its production of the hormone (gonadotrophin releasing hormone) that acts on the pituitary gland. This, in turn, reduces the production of important hormones that act on the ovaries (luteinising hormone and follicle stimulating hormone), causing them to produce less oestrogen and progesterone. The end result is a deficiency of oestrogen and progesterone and a cessation of menstrual periods (*see* fig. 2).

Low body fat levels also upset the metabolism of the sex hormones, reducing their potency and thus fertility. Therefore, a very low body fat level drastically reduces a woman's chances of getting pregnant. However, the good news is that once your body fat level increases over your threshold, your hormonal balance, periods and fertility return to normal.

Figure 2: *The development of amenorrhoea*

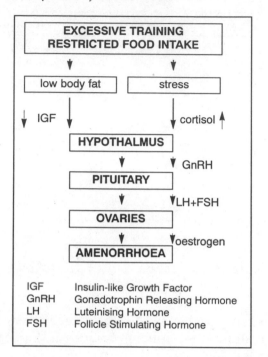

What are the dangers for men of attaining very low body fat levels?

Studies on competitive male wrestlers 'making weight' for contests found that once body fat levels fell below 5%, testosterone levels decreased, causing a drastic fall in sperm count, libido and sexual activity! Studies on male runners found similar changes. Thankfully, though, testosterone levels and libido return to normal once body fat increases. Team doctors in the US now recommend a minimum of 7% fat before allowing wrestlers to compete.

Can a low body fat harm your bones?

Amenorrhoea can lead to more serious problems such as bone loss. That's because low oestrogen levels result in loss of bone minerals and, therefore, bone density (*see* fig. 3). In younger (pre-menopausal) women, this is called *osteopoenia* (i.e. lower bone density than normal for age), which is similar to the osteoporosis that affects post-menopausal women, where bones become thinner, lighter and more fragile. Amenorrhoeic athletes, therefore, run a greater risk of stress fractures. The British Olympic Medical Centre has reported cases of athletes in their 20s and 30s with osteoporotic-type fractures.

Figure 3: *Low body fat and bone density*

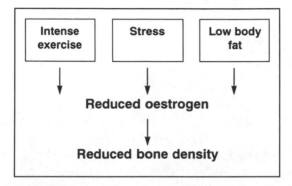

What are the problems with low fat diets?

Very low fat intakes can leave you deficient in a variety of nutrients and lead to several health problems. You will certainly be missing out on the essential fatty acids (linoleic acid and linolenic acid) found in vegetable oils, seeds, nuts and oily fish (*see* page 132), and will therefore be susceptible to dull flaky skin and other dermatological problems; cold extremities; prostaglandin (hormone) imbalance; poor control of inflammation, blood pressure, vasoconstriction and blood clotting.

Low fat diets will be low in fat-soluble vitamins A, D and E. More importantly, fat is needed to enable your body to absorb and transport them, and to convert beta-carotene into vitamin A in the body. Although you can get vitamin D from UV light and vitamin A from its precursor, beta-carotene, in brightly coloured fruit and vegetables, getting enough vitamin E can be much more of a problem. It is found in significant quantities only in vegetable oils, seeds, nuts and egg yolk. Vitamin E is an important antioxidant that protects our cells from harmful free radical attack (*see* Chapter 4). It is thought to help prevent heart disease, certain cancers and even retard aging. It may also help reduce muscle soreness after hard exercise. So, cutting out oils, nuts and seeds means you are increasing your risk of free radical damage.

Chronically low fat diets often result in a low calorie and low nutrient intake overall. Low calorie diets quickly lead to depleted glycogen (carbohydrate) stores, resulting in poor energy levels, reducing capacity for exercise, fatigue, poor recovery between workouts and eventual burn-out. They can also increase protein breakdown – causing loss of muscle mass and strength or a lack of muscular development. This is just the opposite of what you should be achieving in your fitness programme.

How much fat should I eat?

The International Conference on Foods, Nutrition and Sports Performance recommended a healthy fat intake of between 15% and 30% of calories for sportspeople. This is in line with the maximum recommended by the World Health Organisation (30% of calories) and the UK government (33–35% of calories). For the average woman eating 2000 kcal this is equivalent to 33–66 g fat a day. If you eat 2500 kcal, your daily intake should be 42–83 g fat; if you eat 3000 kcal, 50–100 g. Most of your fat intake should come from unsaturated fats, found in vegetable oils (e.g. olive, rapeseed, sunflower), nuts (all kinds), seeds (e.g. sunflower, sesame, pumpkin), oily fish (e.g. sardines, mackerel, salmon), peanut butter and avocado.

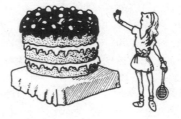

What are fats?

Fats and oils found in food consist mainly of *triglycerides*. These are made up of a unit of glycerol and three fatty acids. Each fatty acid is a chain of carbon and hydrogen atoms with a carboxyl group (-COOH) at one end and a methyl group at the other end (-CH$_3$) – chain lengths between 14 and 22 carbon atoms are most common. These fatty acids are classified in three different groups, according to their chemical structure: saturated, mono-unsaturated and poly-unsaturated. In food, the proportions of each group determine whether the fat is hard or liquid, how it is handled by the body and how it affects your health.

What are saturated fats?

Saturated fatty acids are fully saturated with the maximum amount of hydrogen; in other words, all of their carbon atoms are linked with a single bond to hydrogen atoms. Fats containing a high proportion of saturates are hard at room temperature and mostly come from animal products such as butter, lard, cheese and meat fat. Processed foods made from these fats include biscuits, cakes and pastry. Alternatives to animal fats are palm oil and coconut oil. Also highly saturated, these are often used in margarine, as well as in biscuits and bakery products.

Saturated fatty acids are considered the culprit fat in heart disease because they can increase total cholesterol and the more harmful low density lipoprotein (LDL) cholesterol in the blood. The Department of Health recommend a saturated fatty acid intake of no more than 10% of calories.

What are monounsaturated fats?

Monounsaturated fatty acids have slightly less hydrogen because their carbon chains contain one double or unsaturated bond (hence 'mono'). Oils rich in monounsaturates are usually liquid at room temperature, but may solidify at cold temperatures. The richest sources include olive, rapeseed, groundnut, hazelnut and almond oil, avocados, olives, nuts and seeds.

Monounsaturated fatty acids are thought to have the greatest health benefits. They can reduce total cholesterol, in particular LDL cholesterol, without affecting the beneficial high density lipoprotein (HDL) cholesterol. The Department of Health recommend a monounsaturated fatty acid intake of up to 12% of calories.

What are polyunsaturated fats?

Polyunsaturated fatty acids have the least hydrogen – the carbon chains contain two or more double bonds (hence 'poly'). Oils rich in polyunsaturates are liquid at both room and cold temperatures. Rich sources include most vegetable oils and oily fish (and their oils).

Polyunsaturates can reduce LDL blood cholesterol levels –

however they can also lower the good HDL cholesterol slightly. It is a good idea to replace some with mono-unsaturates, if you eat a lot of them. For this reason, the Department of Health recommend a maximum intake of 10% of calories.

What are the essential fatty acids?

Certain polyunsaturates cannot be made in the body and need to be supplied in the diet. They are called essential fatty acids and are grouped into two series, the n-3 and the n-6 series, derived from linoleic and linolenic acid respectively. The body uses these to make other polyunsaturated fatty acids. The main sources of n-3 fatty acids in the diet include oily fish and their oils, and certain vegetable oils, especially rapeseed, soyabean and linseed oil. The n-6 series of fatty acids are found mainly in vegetable oils, such as corn, sunflower and safflower oil.

The essential fatty acids form a vital part of cell membranes and are converted in the body into hormone-like substances called prostaglandins, thromboxanes and leukotrienes. These control many functions, such as blood clotting, inflammation, the tone of capillary/artery wall muscles, widening and constriction of blood vessels, blood pressure and your immune system. They also help control blood cholesterol levels and blood fat levels. Linoleic acid is important for the skin, helping to make it watertight. People on very low fat diets, deficient in linoleic acid, often develop extremely dry, flaky skin.

The Department of Health recommend that the essential fatty acids (as a sub group of polyunsaturated fatty acids) provide at least 1–2% of calories.

What are trans fatty acids?

Small amounts of trans fatty acids are found naturally in meat and dairy products, but most come from processed fats. These are produced by hydrogenation, a process which changes liquid oils into solid or spreadable fats. During this highly pressurised heat treatment, the geometrical arrangement of the atoms changes. Technically speaking, one or more of the unsaturated double bonds in the fatty acid is altered from the usual *cis* form to the unusual *trans* form. Hydrogenated fats and oils are used in many foods, including cakes, biscuits, margarine, low fat spreads and pastries – check the ingredients.

The exact effect of trans fatty acids on the body is not certain, but it is thought that they may be worse than saturates: they could lower HDL and raise LDL levels. They may also increase levels of a substance that promotes blood clot formation and stops your body using essential fatty acids properly. A US study in 1993 of 85,000 nurses by researchers at Harvard Medical School linked high intakes of trans fatty acids (from processed fats, not natural fats) with a 50% increase in the risk of heart disease. Until more research has been carried out, it is probably best to regard them as similar to saturates and avoid them as far as possible. In practice, this means cutting down on hard margarine (the softer the spread, the fewer trans fatty acids it is likely to contain), fried foods from fast food chains (many use hydrogenated oils), biscuits and other bakery products that contain hydrogenated fats (check the ingredients).

The Department of Health recommend that trans fatty acids make up no more than 2% of calories and that we eat no more than 5 g per day. Unfortunately, they are not normally listed on nutrition labels.

What is cholesterol?

Cholesterol is an essential part of our bodies, making cell membranes and several hormones. Some cholesterol comes from our diet, but most is made in the liver from saturated fats. In fact, the cholesterol we eat has only a small effect on our LDL cholesterol; if we eat more cholesterol (from meat, offal, eggs, dairy products, seafood) the liver compensates by making less, and vice versa. This keeps a steady level of cholesterol in the bloodstream.

Several factors can push up blood cholesterol levels. The major ones are obesity (especially android or central obesity), lack of exercise and the amount of saturated fatty acids we eat. Studies have shown that replacing saturated fatty acids with carbohydrates or unsaturated fatty acids can lower total and LDL cholesterol levels.

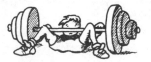

So, which are the best types of fats to eat?

In general, eat all types of fats and oils in moderation – remember, they should make up 15–30% of your total calorie intake. Most people eat considerably more than this (around 41% of calories). Use all spreading fats sparingly – there are advantages and disadvantages with butter, margarine and low fat spreads. Butter, for example, is high in saturated fatty acids but contains no artificial additives. Most margarines and low fat spreads contain trans fatty acids and artificial additives, but are lower in saturates and higher in unsaturates. It really depends on your taste preferences. However, it is best to avoid hard margarines (those which don't spread straight from the fridge) as they have a higher content of hydrogenated fats and trans fatty acids.

For cooking and salad dressings, choose oils which are high in monounsaturated fatty acids – olive, rapeseed and nut oils are good choices for health as well as taste. Include small amounts of nuts and seeds in your regular diet; they provide many valuable nutrients apart from monounsaturates. If you eat fish, include one to two portions of oily fish (e.g. mackerel, herring, salmon) per week.

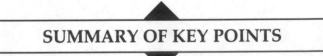

SUMMARY OF KEY POINTS

- Excess body fat is a disadvantage in almost all sports and fitness programmes, reducing power, speed and performance.
- Very low body fat does not guarantee improved performance either. There appears to be an optimal fat range for each individual which cannot be predicted by a standard linear relationship.
- There are three main components of body fat: essential fat (for tissue structure); sex specific fat (for hormonal function); and storage fat (for energy).
- The minimum percentage of fat recommended for men is 5% and for women, 10%. However, for normal health, the recommended ranges are 13–18% and 18–25% respectively. In practice, many athletes fall below these recommended ranges.
- Very low body fat levels are associated with hormonal imbalance

(in both sexes), amenorrhoea, infertility, reduced bone density and increased risk of osteoporosis.

- Very low fat diets can lead to deficient intakes of essential fatty acids and fat soluble vitamins. In the long term, fat and calorie restriction can result in other nutritional imbalances, depleted glycogen stores, chronic fatigue, loss of lean tissue and reduced performance.
- A fat intake of 15–30% of energy is recommended for athletes and active people.
- Unsaturated fatty acids should make up the majority of the fat intake, with saturated fatty acids and trans fatty acids kept to a minimum.

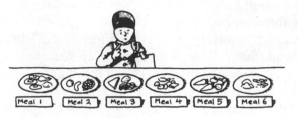

8

Weight management

Many athletes and fitness participants wish to lose or gain weight, whether for health or performance reasons, or in order to make a competitive weight category. However, rapid weight loss can have serious health consequences leading to a marked reduction in performance. A knowledge of safe weight loss methods is, therefore, essential. Since 95% of dieters fail to maintain their weight loss within a five year period, lifestyle management is the key to long term weight management.

This chapter examines the effects of weight loss on performance and health, and highlights the dangers of rapid weight loss methods. It examines the reasons why many people find it hard to lose and maintain weight, and the barriers to long term success. New research on appetite control and metabolism is presented, along with the dangers of 'yo-yo dieting' or weight cycling. It explodes many of the myths and fallacies about metabolic rate and, finally, gives safe and simple step-by-step strategies for successful weight loss and weight gain.

Will dieting affect my performance?

Many athletes believe that losing weight improves their chances of winning but, in practice, rapid or strict dieting can have an adverse effect on your performance.

Firstly, rapid weight loss results in a diminished aerobic capacity. A drop of up to 5% has been measured in athletes who had lost just 2–3% of body weight through dehydration. A loss of 10% can occur in those who lose weight through strict dieting.

Anaerobic performance, strength and muscular endurance are also decreased, although researchers have found that strength (expressed against body weight) can actually improve after gradual weight loss. Strict dieting also reduces vitamin and mineral status, since a lower food intake almost always means a lower intake of micronutrients. Supplements may, therefore, be advisable if dieting for more than three weeks.

Prolonged dieting or food restriction can have more serious health consequences. In female athletes, low body weight and body fat have been linked with menstrual irregularities, amenorrhoea and stress fractures; in male athletes, with reduced testosterone production. It has also been suggested that the combination of intense training, food restriction and the psychological pressure for extreme leanness may precipitate disordered eating and clinical eating disorders in some athletes. Scientists say that those who attempt to lose body fat for appearance are more likely to develop an eating disorder than those who control it only for performance purposes.

Rapid weight loss

To make weight for a competition (e.g. boxing, bodybuilding, judo), athletes may resort to rapid weight loss methods, such as fasting, dehydration, exercising in sweat suits, saunas, diet pills, laxatives, diuretics or self induced vomiting. Weight losses of 10 lb in 3 days are not uncommon. In one study [1] of 180 female athletes, 32% admitted they used more than one of these methods. In another [2], 15% of young female swimmers said they had tried one of these methods.

1 L.W. Rosen et al., *Physician and Sportsmed* (14,79–86, 1986)
2 G.M. Drummer et al., *Physician and Sportsmed* (15,75–85, 1987)

What happens to the body during rapid weight loss?

Rapid weight loss inevitably leads to dehydration and glycogen depletion. This causes a reduced cardiac output and stroke volume, reduced plasma volume, slower nutrient exchange and slower waste removal, all of which have an impact on health and performance. In moderately intense exercise lasting more than 30 seconds, even dehydration of less than 5% body weight will diminish strength or performance, although it does not appear to affect exercise lasting less than 30 seconds. So, for athletes relying on pure strength (e.g. weight lifting), rapid weight loss may not be as detrimental.

Will I still be able to train hard whilst losing weight?

You should still have plenty of energy to train hard provided you do not restrict your carbohydrate intake. One consistent finding from studies is that a high carbohydrate intake (at least 60% of energy) is critical for preserving muscular endurance, and both aerobic and anaerobic capacity. A lower than optimal intake results in glycogen depletion and increased protein oxidation. Researchers recommend that a protein intake of approximately 1.6 g/ kg body weight/day is necessary to maintain body protein and muscle mass during weight loss. The normal requirement for sedentary individuals is 0.75 g/kg; for athletes, 1.2–1.7 g/kg. It is also recommended that weight loss should not exceed 1.0 kg/ week.

Exercise scientists now recommend reference to body fat *ranges* rather than *optimal values*, as the optimal body fat for performance and appearance are not necessarily the same. Consequently, an athlete may achieve the desirable appearance, but to the detriment of his or her performance. There is actually little evidence that attaining a certain body fat/weight automatically improves an athlete's performance; genetic endowment, strenuous training and good nutrition appear to be the main reasons for success.

Most weight loss methods, particularly those which result in dehydration and glycogen depletion, will have a detrimental effect on performance. Assess your training goals carefully and accept that a reduction in body fat may not necessarily solve your problems. Any weight loss programme should be gradual; aim to lose 0.5–1 kg per week; a calorie intake of no less than 25 kcal/kg body weight should achieve this. Your diet should consist of at least 60% carbohydrate calories, 15–25% fat and 15–20% protein. Finally, avoid dieting altogether during periods of intense training.

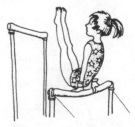

How can I lose body fat?

To lose body fat, you have to expend more energy (calories) than you consume. In other words, you have to achieve a negative energy balance (*see* fig. 1).

Figure 1: *Energy balance equations*

Energy Balance		
Energy intake (Food and Drink)	=	*Energy expenditure* (Basal metabolism, dietary thermogenesis, physical activity)
Positive Energy Balance		
Energy intake (Food and Drink)	>	*Energy expenditure* (Basal metabolism, dietary thermogenesis, physical activity)
Negative Energy Balance		
Energy intake (Food and Drink)	<	*Energy expenditure* (Basal metabolism, dietary thermogenesis, physical activity)
(< = less than, > = more than)		

Research has shown that a combination of diet and activity is more likely to result in long term success than diet or exercise alone. Unfortunately, there are no miracle solutions or short cuts. The objectives of a healthy diet and exercise programme are to:

- achieve a modest negative energy (calorie) balance
- maintain (or even increase) lean tissue
- gradually reduce body fat percentage
- avoid a significant reduction in basal metabolic rate
- maintain a high percentage energy from carbohydrate (60%) and a low percentage from fat (15–25%)
- achieve an optimal intake of vitamins and minerals.

Step 1: Set realistic goals

Before embarking on a weight loss plan, write down your goals clearly, as research has proven that by writing down your intentions, you are far more likely to turn them into actions.

These goals should be specific, positive and realistic ('I will lose 14 lb of body fat') rather than hopeful ('I would like to lose some weight'). Try to allow a suitable time frame (*see* Step 3): to lose 3 stone one month before a summer holiday is, obviously, unrealistic! Make sure, also, that you are clear about your reasons for wanting to lose weight: many normal-weight women wrongly believe that losing weight will solve their emotional or body image problems.

Step 2: Monitor body composition changes

The best way to monitor your progress is by a combination of simple girth or circumference measurements (e.g. chest, waist, hips, arms, legs), as in Figure 2, and by skinfold thickness measurements, obtained by calipers. Exercise physiologists recommend keeping a record of the skinfold thickness measurements themselves rather than converting them into body fat percentages. This is because the conversion charts are based on equations for the average, sedentary person and may not be appropriate for sportspeople or very lean or fat individuals. The

Figure 2: Girth measurements

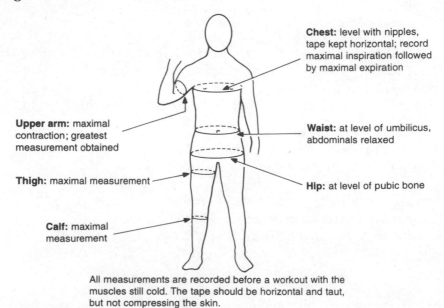

Chest: level with nipples, tape kept horizontal; record maximal inspiration followed by maximal expiration

Upper arm: maximal contraction; greatest measurement obtained

Waist: at level of umbilicus, abdominals relaxed

Thigh: maximal measurement

Hip: at level of pubic bone

Calf: maximal measurement

All measurements are recorded before a workout with the muscles still cold. The tape should be horizontal and taut, but not compressing the skin.

same argument applies to several other methods of body fat measurement, such as bio-electrical impedence and near-infra-red interactance. Monitoring changes in measurements at specific sites of the body allows you to see how your shape is changing and where most fat is being lost. This is a far better motivator than weighing scales!

Step 3: Aim to lose 1–2 lb fat per week

Weekly or fortnightly weighing can be useful for checking the speed of weight/fat loss, but do not rely exclusively on this method as it does not reflect changes in body composition! Avoid more frequent weighing as this can lead to an obsession with weight. Bear in mind that weight loss in the first week may be as much as 5 lb, but this is mostly glycogen and its accompanying fluid (1 lb glycogen is stored with up to 4 lb water). Afterwards, aim to lose no more than 2 lb fat per week. Faster weight loss usually suggests a loss of lean tissue, so you should increase your calorie intake by 250–500 per day to slow it down to a healthy level.

Step 4: Keep a food diary

A food diary is a written record of your daily food and drink intake. It is a very good way to evaluate your present eating habits and to find out exactly what, why and when you are eating. It will allow you to check whether your diet is well balanced or lacking in any important nutrients, and to take a more careful look at your usual meal patterns and lifestyle.

Weigh and write down everything you eat and drink for at least three consecutive days – ideally seven. This period should include at least one weekend day. It is important not to change your usual diet at this time! Every spoonful of sugar in tea, every scrape of butter on bread should be recorded (*see* Table 1).

Step 5: Estimate calorie, carbohydrate, fat and protein intake

You can carry out a basic dietary analysis with the help of a food composition book such as McCance & Widdowson's *Composition of Foods* (available through HMSO). To calculate the percentage of energy from carbohydrate, fat and protein, consult Table 2, then compare with the recommendations.

Table 1: *Sample food diary*

Time	Where	With whom	Food/drink	Quantity
7.30 am	Kitchen	Alone	Orange juice Toast (white) Butter Marmalade Tea with semi- skimmed milk	1 glass 2 slices 2 tsp 4 tsp 1 cup
11 am	Office	Friends	Coffee with semi- skimmed milk Doughnut	1 large mug 1
1 pm	Pub	Friends	Ploughman's: French bread Butter Cheese Coleslaw Pickle Lager	 6″ piece 2 pats approx. 3 oz 2 tbsp 1 tbsp 1 pint
6 pm	Kitchen	Alone	Digestive biscuits Coffee with semi- skimmed milk	4 1 mug
7.30 pm	Dining room	Family	Fried sausages Chips Peas Lager Ice cream	2 small 8 oz 2 tbsp 1 pint 2 scoops
9.30 pm	Lounge	Husband	Coffee with semi- skimmed milk Chocolates Baileys	1 cup 3 oz 2 glasses
Exercise	Walked to tube station – 10 min Walked to pub – 5 min Walked from tube station – 10 min Aerobics class – 45 min			

Table 2: *To calculate % energy*

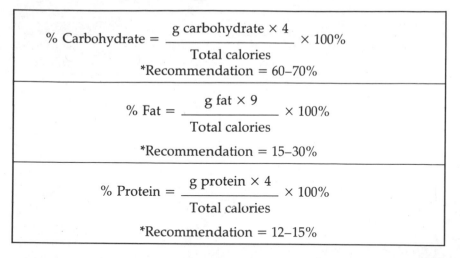

$$\% \text{ Carbohydrate} = \frac{\text{g carbohydrate} \times 4}{\text{Total calories}} \times 100\%$$

*Recommendation = 60–70%

$$\% \text{ Fat} = \frac{\text{g fat} \times 9}{\text{Total calories}} \times 100\%$$

*Recommendation = 15–30%

$$\% \text{ Protein} = \frac{\text{g protein} \times 4}{\text{Total calories}} \times 100\%$$

*Recommendation = 12–15%

* *Food, Nutrition and Sports Performance – Proceedings of an International Scientific Consensus* (Journal of Sports Science, Summer 1991)

Step 6: Cut calories slowly

To lose 1 lb fat a week, aim to create a calorie deficit of 3500 kcal a week or approximately 500 per day. The most effective way is by increasing energy expenditure *and* decreasing energy intake. So, for example, if your normal intake is 2500 kcal per day, you could reduce your calorie intake to 2200 kcal and increase energy expenditure by 200 kcal (e.g. 45 minute walk). That is equivalent to a 500 kcal deficit per day. If fat loss slows down or reaches a plateau, reduce calorie intake slightly further or increase the intensity, frequency or duration of your exercise programme.

Step 7: Never consume fewer calories than your BMR

Calorie intake should never be less than your basal metabolic rate (*see* Table 3), otherwise you risk losing excessive lean tissue, severely depleting your glycogen stores and having an inadequate nutrient intake. In practice, most people should be able to lose weight eating 1500–2000 kcal per day, especially if they increase their activity level. It is erroneous and potentially dangerous to prescribe low calorie diets of 1000 kcal or less.

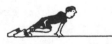

Table 3: *How to estimate your BMR*

Men		Women	
Weight (kg)	BMR (kcal/day)	Weight (kg)	BMR (kcal/day)
70	1680	50	1250
75	1730	55	1290
80	1790	60	1330
85	1850	65	1370
90	1910	70	1410
95	1960	75	1450
100	2020	80	1500

Step 8: Trim the fat

Look carefully at your food diary and identify the high fat foods that you are currently eating. Aim to reduce intake to 15–25% by making lower fat substitutions – check Table 4 for suggestions. Remember, don't try to cut fat out completely, as we need the equivalent of 1 tablespoon of oil (or 1 oz nuts or seeds) per day to get our quota of essential fatty acids and vitamin E.

No food should be banned completely or regarded as taboo – this could lead to an obsessive and negative attitude towards food, which is psychologically harmful in the long term. All foods are allowable – it's the frequency and amounts that need watching!

Step 9: Eat more frequently

Plan to eat at least 4–6 times a day, planning snacks and meals at regular intervals. This does not mean increasing the amount eaten, rather eating moderate sized meals or snacks more frequently. Research has shown that each time we eat, the metabolic rate increases approximately 10% for a short while afterwards. This phenomenon is the *thermic* effect of food, or dietary-induced thermogenesis, and is roughly equivalent to the extra energy cost of digesting, absorbing, transporting and metabolising the food. Researchers have also found that frequent eating keeps blood sugar and insulin levels more stable, as well as helping to control blood cholesterol levels. For regular exercisers, eating six times a day is especially beneficial for speedy glycogen (carbohydrate) replenishment between workouts, and for minimising fat deposition. A regular food intake also ensures a constant flux of nutrients for repairing body tissues.

Table 4: Trim the fat

Eat less of the following:
(These foods are high in fat but relatively low in other essential nutrients.)

- butter, margarine and other spreading fats
- fried foods
- fatty meats and processed meat products (e.g. sausages, burgers, meat pies)
- pastry dishes
- cakes, biscuits, puddings
- chocolate
- crisps and similar potato/corn/wheat snacks.

Make the following substitutions:
(These foods provide some fat together with other essential nutrients.)

- semi-skimmed or skimmed milk instead of full fat milk
- low fat spread or peanut butter instead of butter or margarine
- low or reduced fat cheese instead of ordinary cheese
- jacket or boiled potatoes instead of chips
- chicken, fish or lean meat instead of fatty meat, burgers and sausages
- crackers, rice cakes or fruit bars instead of biscuits and cakes
- fresh fruit instead of chocolate.

Make the following changes:
(These will reduce your fat intake while supplying other essential nutrients.)

- limit frying to stir frying with minimal amounts of oil
- top baked potatoes with fromage frais, yoghurt, half fat creme fraiche or baked beans
- remove skin from chicken or turkey
- grill, bake, stir fry or boil instead of frying
- make low fat salad dressings with flavoured vinegar (e.g. raspberry); yoghurt seasoned with fresh herbs, lemon or lime juice; fromage frais seasoned with mustard
- choose lean cuts of meat and trim off as much fat as possible.

Table 5: *Low fat snack ideas*

- Sandwiches, rolls, pitta, bagels with low fat fillings, e.g. banana, cottage cheese, tuna, chicken, salad
- English muffins, fruit buns, scones
- Potato scones or farls
- Breadsticks, popcorn, pretzels
- Oat/Scotch/homemade pancakes
- Oatcakes and rice cakes with low fat toppings, e.g. banana, fruit spread
- Toast with honey, fruit spread or baked beans
- Fresh fruit, e.g. bananas, apples, pears, grapes
- Dried fruit, e.g. raisins, apricots, dates, apple rings
- Dried fruit bars, some cereal bars
- Home made shakes made with low fat milk, fruit and yoghurt
- Low fat yoghurt, fromage frais

Step 10: Make gradual lifestyle changes

Long term weight management can be achieved with healthy eating and regular exercise. However, one of the biggest barriers to this is an unwillingness to commit to a few necessary changes in lifestyle. Table 6 lists some of the common reasons why many people fail to manage their weight in the long term, together with some suggestions as to how to overcome them.

What is the best way to make weight for my competition?

Certain sports, such as boxing, judo, lightweight rowing and bodybuilding, require athletes to compete at a particular weight. Losing weight to meet class requirements is called 'making weight'. For weight matched competitions, it is an advantage to be as close as possible to the upper limit of your weight category. However, this should not be achieved at the expense of losing lean tissue (by rapid severe dieting), depleting your glycogen stores (by starving) or dehydration (by saunas, sweat suits, diuretics or restricting fluids).

Table 6: *Lifestyle changes*

Excuse	Suggestion
Not enough time to prepare healthy meals	Plan meals in advance so all ingredients are at hand. Make meals in bulk and refrigerate/freeze portions. Cook baked potatoes, pasta and rice in larger quantities and save.
Work shifts	Plan regular snack breaks and take own food with you.
Work involves lots of travelling	Take portable snacks, e.g. rolls, fruit, energy bars, muffins, dried fruit, fruit juice (diluted).
Need to cook for rest of family	Adapt favourite family meals, e.g. spaghetti bolognese, to contain less fat, more carbohydrate and fibre (e.g. leaner mince, more vegetables, wholemeal pasta). Make meals that everyone enjoys.
Overeat when stressed	Consider stress counselling or relaxation courses to learn to handle stressful situations; take up new sport/hobby/leisure interests.
Eat out frequently	Choose lower fat, higher carbohydrate meals in restaurants, e.g. pasta with vegetable sauces, chicken tikka with chappati, stir fried vegetables with rice.

The principles for making weight for competition are similar to those for weight loss. In summary:

◆ Set a realistic and achievable goal.
◆ Allow enough time – aim to lose 1–2 lb (0.5–1 kg) body fat per week.

- Monitor your weight and body composition by skinfold thickness measurements and girth measurements.
- Reduce your calorie intake by 250–500 kcal per day – never eat less than your basal metabolic rate.
- Increase the amount/frequency of aerobic training.
- Maintain carbohydrate intake at 60–70% of calories.
- Reduce fat intake to 15–25% of calories.
- Maintain protein intake at 1.2–1.7g/kg/day.
- Eat at frequent, regular intervals (5–6 times a day).

Avoid losing weight at the last minute by starvation or dehydration, as this can be dangerous. Starvation leads to depleted glycogen stores, so you will not be able to perform at your best. Dehydration leads to electrolyte disturbances, cramp and heartbeat irregularities. It is unlikely that you will be able to refuel and rehydrate sufficiently between the weigh-in and your competition, so aim to be at or within your weight category at least a day before the weigh-in.

If you find it very difficult to make weight without resorting to these dangerous methods, consider competing in the next weight category.

Should I count calories?

Calorie counting does not give you the full picture. Although you need to be in a negative energy balance to lose weight, new research suggests that the total number of calories is less important than the relative amounts of fat, carbohydrate and protein in your diet; calories from each of these sources are handled by the body in quite different ways. This, in turn, has an important bearing on body fat levels. Scientists are now looking at the separate balance equations for each macronutrient.

Can alcohol make you fat?

Indirectly, alcohol can encourage fat storage. Since alcohol cannot be stored in the body, it must be oxidised and converted into energy (*see* Chapter 6). Whilst this is happening, the oxidation of fat and carbohydrate is suppressed, and these are channelled into storage instead.

Alcohol provides 7 kcal/g, which can significantly increase your total calorie intake if you consume large quantities. Also, many alcoholic drinks contain sugars and other carbohydrates, which increase the calorie content further.

Can protein make you fat?

When protein is overeaten, the amino part of the molecule is excreted and the remainder of the molecule provides an energy substrate. This can either be used directly for energy production or else stored – preferably as glycogen rather than fat. Furthermore, protein ingestion actually stimulates protein oxidation, so a significant proportion of the protein calories are given off as heat.

The result is that, for most people, the amount of protein in the body (muscle, organ tissue, blood proteins, etc.) remains relatively constant. It only increases in response to growth stimuli (e.g. during childhood and adolescence), strength training or certain hormones, and is, therefore, unlikely to be 'fattening' unless grossly overeaten.

Can carbohydrate make you fat?

Although possible in theory, in practice it is relatively difficult for the body to convert surplus carbohydrate calories into fat. Carbohydrate that is surplus to the body's immediate needs is stored as glycogen or given off as heat. As with protein, studies have shown that when carbohydrate is overeaten, carbohydrate oxidation increases. In other words, some of the carbohydrate is burned off and effectively wasted as heat. As much as 23% of the calories from carbohydrate are lost through this route, and the rest is preferably converted into glycogen.

Can fat make you fat?

Dietary fat is far more likely to make you fat than any other nutrient, as it is stored as adipose (fat) tissue if not required straight away. In contrast to carbohydrate and protein, overeating fat does not increase fat oxidation; this only occurs when total energy demands exceed total energy intake or during aerobic exercise.

Fat contains more than double the calories per gram (9 kcal/g) of carbohydrate and protein (both 4 kcal/g), but it is much easier to overconsume as it is less satiating for two reasons. Firstly, carbohydrate and protein produce a rise in blood glucose, which reduces the appetite. Fat, on the other hand, is digested and absorbed less rapidly, and often actually depresses blood glucose, thereby failing to satisfy the appetite as efficiently. Secondly, fatty foods usually have a high calorie density and low bulk, again making them less satisfying, even in the short term, and easier to overeat.

Fat makes you fat

The hypothesis that fat is more fattening, calorie for calorie, than carbohydrate, is supported by a number of well controlled studies. In a study of prisoners at Vermont, it was found that lean men gained weight more readily when overfed calories on a high fat diet than on a mixed diet of carbohydrate and fat. In another recent study, men were fed 150% of their calorie requirements for two 14-day periods. In one period, the excess calories came from fat; in the other, from carbohydrate. Overfeeding fat caused much greater deposition of body fat than overfeeding carbohydrate. What's more, this effect was magnified in the obese men.

What is the key to appetite control?

It appears that carbohydrate plays a key role in regulating our appetite and thus in achieving long term weight control. Carbohydrate is stored as glycogen in the liver and muscles. Any fluctuations in our glycogen stores are detected by our appetite control centre in the brain and translated into feelings of hunger. So, when glycogen stores are low, we experience an increased appetite and eat more. When glycogen stores are full, our appetite is reduced and we eat less. Therefore, it is much harder to gain body fat when eating a high carbohydrate, low fat diet.

What is an 'adipostat'?

Scientists have identified a gene which acts as an *adipostat*, controlling body fat levels. It is set to a particular fat level, so when body fat levels change, the adipostat changes our metabolic rate and appetite in order to restore our body fat level. For example, if body fat levels drop too low (e.g. after prolonged dieting), the adipostat reduces the metabolic rate and increases appetite. If body fat levels increase too far, the adipostat increases the metabolic rate and reduces appetite.

High carbohydrate diets and appetite control

Researchers at the Dunn Clinical Nutrition Centre in Cambridge fed volunteers one of three identical-looking diets containing either 60%, 40% or 20% fat calories. Those who consumed the 20% fat diet either maintained or lost body fat after seven days. Those who consumed the higher fat diets gained up to 0.9 kg body fat. None of the volunteers were aware of the fat content of their food, nor of the purpose of the experiment. All felt equally satisfied on their diet.

Experiments at the Human Appetite and Research Unit in Leeds found that volunteers who consumed a high carbohydrate, low fat breakfast experienced less hunger for several hours afterwards than those who had eaten a higher fat breakfast of equal calories. Both breakfasts looked identical, so volunteers did not know the fat content of their meal. They were asked to keep a food diary for the rest of the day. Those who had consumed the higher fat breakfast went on to eat 800 more calories than those who had eaten the low fat, high carbohydrate breakfast.

What are the practical implications?

It is important to dispel the myth about carbohydrates being fattening. In fact, it is almost impossible to become fat on a high carbohydrate, low fat diet. Beware, rather, of high fat foods, which are easily overeaten, resulting in a positive energy balance, and remember that dietary fat is more likely to be deposited as body fat at a lower metabolic cost than for other nutrients. Therefore, the cornerstone of long term, successful weight control is a low fat, high carbohydrate diet. If you eat until your appetite is satisfied and stick to low fat foods, body fat levels will automatically be controlled.

Do overweight people have a slow metabolism?

Unfortunately, there's no truth is this theory whatsoever. It is very easy to blame an inability to lose weight or sustain weight loss on a sluggish metabolism. Many studies have demonstrated that basal metabolic rate (BMR) tends to be proportional to total body weight. In other words, the heavier you are, the higher your BMR. Standard equations for predicting BMR from body weight are published by the World Health Organisation (*see* Table 3). Obviously, as your weight decreases by dieting, your BMR will decrease proportionally but, for most dieters, the difference is relatively insignificant. For example, if your weight decreased from 75 kg to 65 kg (i.e. a weight loss of 10 kg), your BMR would drop a mere 80 kcal. In other words, you would need to consume 80 calories less per day to sustain your new weight.

Therefore, except in a few very rare cases (e.g. hypothyroidism, Cushing's Syndrome), there is no truth in the slow metabolism theory, or in the belief that having a sluggish metabolism makes it impossible to lose weight.

Table 7: *Finding your total daily expenditure (calories needed to maintain weight)*

Inactive	Moderately active	Active
very inactive occupation; sitting most of day; no sport/exercise	inactive occupation; light activity at home; occasional sport/exercise	active occupation *or* regular strenuous exercise/sport *or* daily walking/cycling
1.3 × BMR	**1.5 × BMR**	**1.7 × BMR**

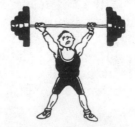

Does dieting make me burn calories more slowly than before?

A lighter body expends fewer calories for any given activity than a heavier body (one of the basic laws of physics!), so as you lose weight, you will burn fewer calories. But, there are other far more important factors (such as exercise intensity, duration and your fitness level) which can affect your total energy expenditure.

For example, if you weigh 75 kg, you will burn 232 kcal during 30 minutes of medium intensity aerobics. If you weigh 65 kg, you will burn 201 kcal during the same period of time: a relatively small drop of 31 kcal. However, at 65 kg, if you increase the intensity of the aerobics, then you will burn considerably more calories (263 kcal). If you extend your exercise session to 45 minutes, you will burn even more (395 kcal!). So, to burn more calories and fat, increase your exercise time and intensity rather than worry about your weight.

Exercise and Calorie Burning

Researchers at the Dunn Clinical Nutrition Centre in Cambridge measured the energy expenditure in lean and obese people during cycling and stepping. In the cycling experiment (a non weight-bearing activity), there was no significant difference in energy costs. However, in the stepping experiment (which *was* a weight-bearing activity), the obese people actually burned more calories than the lean people.

Will dieting lower my metabolic rate?

When you restrict your calorie intake, your BMR slows down a little. This is your body's attempt to conserve energy because it assumes food is in short supply. However, this decrease in BMR is only temporary and is not as much as you may think (usually around 10%, though as much as 30% for severe calorie restriction). The more severe the calorie drop, the greater the drop in BMR. So, to minimise a decrease in your BMR:

♦ reduce your calorie intake as modestly and gradually as possible and also . . .

◆ include regular aerobic and resistance exercise. All exercise increases your energy expenditure and causes a short term rise in BMR, the so-called 'afterburn' or 'excess post-exercise oxygen consumption' (EPOC). Resistance exercise increases lean body tissue, which burns calories even at rest.

For example, if you normally eat 2500 kcal/day, cut down to between 2000 and 2250 kcal, and increase your energy expenditure by around 250 kcal per day. This will result in a calorie deficit of 3500–4750 kcal per week, equivalent to a fat loss of 1–1.5 lb per week. If your weight loss slows, you can gradually cut down to 1750 kcal or increase your energy output. That way you will avoid or at least minimise a drop in your BMR.

In any case, your BMR per kg body weight returns to normal within a week or so as your body adjusts to the new calorie intake. Once you stop dieting and increase your calorie intake, there is actually a small increase in BMR. Therefore, it is a myth that dieting slows down your metabolism in the long term.

Does yo-yo dieting wreck your metabolism?

Many life-long dieters believe that repeated dieting and weight regain (weight cycling) makes the body so efficient at conserving energy that it permanently slows their BMR. The theory is that the body adapts to survive on fewer and fewer calories so that when the diet fails, the body stores fat more readily, making it harder to lose weight next time.

However, there is no scientific data to support this theory. When you restrict your food intake, your BMR falls initially, but soon returns to its original level once normal eating is resumed. A study carried out at the Dunn Clinical Nutrition Centre followed 11 overweight women through three dieting cycles and found that, although their BMR decreased initially, it did not change significantly overall.

Is yo-yo dieting harmful?

Repeated weight fluctuations have been linked with an increased risk of heart disease, secondary diabetes, gall bladder disease and premature death. However, researchers are divided as to the exact reason. One explanation is that fat tends to be redeposited intra-abdominally, closer to the liver, rather than in the peripheral regions of the body, such as the hips, thighs and arms, thus posing a greater heart disease risk. Another explanation is that repeated severe dieting can lead to a loss of lean tissue (including organ tissue) and nutritional deficiencies that can damage heart muscle. Yo-yo dieting can also be bad for your psychological health. Each time you regain weight, you experience a sense of failure, which can lower your confidence and self esteem.

Why does my weight soar once I stop dieting?

There are two main explanations as to why some people gain a lot of weight after dieting. Firstly, many dieters tend to overeat or binge after 'coming off' their diet, especially on foods regarded as forbidden. You are likely, therefore, to consume a lot more calories than before. Researchers say that this is because inappropriate dieting suppresses your natural appetite control and lowers your self esteem, leading to negative moods and exaggerated appetite once you stop dieting. The second explanation is that your glycogen stores simply fill out. Since you store about 4 lb water for every 1 lb glycogen, the scales may register a larger weight gain than expected. Obviously, this is not fat weight, so don't feel disheartened!

So why can't I lose weight?

Many people insist that they hardly eat a thing, yet cannot shift any surplus weight. Clearly, this is impossible. An alternative explanation can usually be found by delving more closely into daily eating habits, lifestyle and psychology. Keeping a detailed, honest, weighed food diary, ideally for seven days, can reveal many truths. Here are some of the most common explanations for 'resistant obesity':

1 Underestimating food intake

Researchers say that many 'resistant' dieters underestimate their food intake. Numerous studies have found that such people consciously or subconsciously underestimate how much they eat. In a study carried out by researchers from the University of Ulster and the Dunn Clinical Nutrition Centre, 16 men and 16 women kept a 7-day, weighed-food diary, while their total energy expenditure was simultaneously measured, using the highly accurate doubly-labelled water method. There was little difference in energy expenditure, but there was a wide variation in reported energy intakes. This discrepancy between energy expenditure and apparent low intakes in some people could only be explained by under-reporting of food intake and not, say the researchers, to any defect in energy metabolism.

2 Weekend splurging

Many people restrict their food intake during the week, then relax restraint at the weekend, celebrating their dieting efforts by splurging on high fat 'treats' – often aided by alcohol. A rigid daily diet of around 1000–1200 kcal from Monday to Friday, can give way to mounting hunger by Friday night, and to a much larger consumption of food over the weekend – perhaps 3000 kcal a day. Despite weekday dieting efforts, the total weekly calorie intake ends up exactly the same as a normal, daily maintenance calorie intake (i.e. non-diet).

Guilt after the weekend splurge brings on renewed resolve to diet more strictly during the coming week. This, again, is followed by hunger, increased appetite, overeating, guilt, and so the vicious circle continues. It is easy to see how the weekday dieter becomes more and more frustrated: he or she feels always on a diet, yet never losing any weight.

3 Daytime starving/evening bingeing

It is common to find that many dieters eat very little during the day, skipping breakfast and surviving only on snacks. Daytime starvation leads to depleted glycogen stores which inevitably leads to exaggerated hunger by the evening and consequent overeating.

A study published in 1993 in the American Journal of Clinical Nutrition found that if you eat in the early part of the day, you burn off more calories by a process called *dietary induced thermogenesis* (DIT), in which energy is used up as a result of digesting and absorbing a meal. Volunteers were given a 544 kcal meal either at 9 am, 5 pm or 1 am. DIT raised calorie expenditure by 16%, 13½%

and 11% respectively. Thus, eating late at night burns off fewer calories than eating during the daytime.

4 Evening nibbles

A food diary may reveal that a dieter's evening meal extends to an all night sitting. It is easy to discount snacks and nibbles consumed mindlessly in front of the television. Many dieters will snack in the evening through boredom, misery, anger or other emotional reasons, without consciously realising or admitting how much they have eaten.

5 Setting an unrealistic goal

Aiming for an unrealistically low body weight is a very common mistake. One theory is that we have a genetically determined 'set point' close to which the body attempts to regulate its weight and body fat. It uses a variety of adaptive mechanisms: studies have shown that when people are underfed, the body reduces its spontaneous physical activity, its thermic response to food (DIT) and, temporarily, its BMR, in response to what the body perceives as imminent starvation. Research by Dr Stunkard in the USA suggests that everyone's body is programmed to be at a certain weight. So, people who are constantly striving to attain a low body weight may be fighting a losing battle with their genes, as well as putting their health at risk and creating unnecessary psychological stress.

6 Dieting mentality

There is evidence that a psychological difference exists between dieters and non-dieters. In dieters and weight conscious people, the normal regulation of food intake becomes undermined as normal appetite and hunger cues are ignored. This leads to periods of restraint and semi starvation, followed by overindulgence and guilt, followed by restraint, and so on.

The psychology of dieting

Dieters usually live by a set of rules centred around allowed foods and banned ('naughty') foods. For example, in one US study, dieters were given two apples (100 kcal) or two squares of chocolate (100 kcal). Those who ate the chocolate perceived themselves to be breaking their diet and went on to overindulge at the subsequent meal. Those who ate the apples continued with their diet.

At the University of Toronto, dieters and non-dieters were given a high calorie milkshake, followed by free access to icecream. The dieters actually went on to eat more icecream than the non-dieters. This is due to a phenomenon known as 'counter regulation'; having lost the inbuilt regulation system of non-dieters, they were unable to detect and thus compensate for the calorie pre-load.

More recently, Dr Barbara Rolls at Penn State University demonstrated that weight worriers appear to lack the internal 'calorie counter' possessed by people who don't worry about their weight. When given a yoghurt half an hour before lunch, those who worried about their weight ate more for lunch than the free and easy people. It appears that such dieters have poor appetite control and are unable to compensate for previous food intake.

Psychologists have shown that habitual dieters tend to have a more emotional personality than those who are not preoccupied with weight. They also tend to be more obsessive and less able to concentrate.

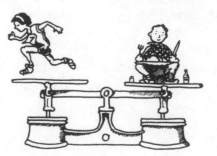

Checklist

- Keep a food diary for a week, writing down the weight of everything you normally eat and drink. This helps you become aware of your true eating pattern.
- Do not skip meals or starve yourself during the day.
- Plan regular meals and snacks throughout the day, thereby eliminating excessive hunger, satisfying appetite, facilitating efficient glycogen refuelling, improving energy levels and health.
- Set yourself a realistic weight goal that is right for your body type.
- Avoid weekday dieting and weekend splurging. Aim to eat about the same amount of food each day and don't worry if you occasionally overdo it.
- Remember, there are no banned foods; all foods are allowed.
- Do not set yourself rigid eating and exercising rules. Be flexible and never feel guilty if you overindulge or miss an exercise session.
- Examine your feelings and emotions when you eat. Food should not be used as a shield for emotional problems. Solve these with the help of a trained counsellor or eating disorder specialist.

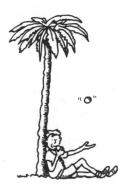

SUMMARY OF KEY POINTS

- Rapid weight loss can result in excessive loss of lean tissue and a reduction in aerobic capacity, strength, muscle endurance and dehydration.
- Prolonged dieting or food restriction can lead to menstrual irregularities and amenorrhoea in women; reduced testosterone production in men; increased risk of stress fractures and bone loss; chronic fatigue; and disordered eating.
- Safe weight loss may be achieved by maintaining a high carbohydrate diet (60%), an adequate protein intake (15–20%), and a low fat intake (15–25%), together with an appropriate exercise programme.
- The recommended rate of weight loss is 0.5–1 kg per week.
- To make weight for a competition, it is essential to set a realistic goal and allow sufficient time to achieve it.
- A high carbohydrate, low fat diet is the key to appetite control and long term weight management.
- BMR is proportional to body weight: there is no evidence that the BMR is reduced in overweight people.
- Food restriction causes only a temporary reduction in BMR, but this may be offset by exercise and, in any case, is restored once normal eating is resumed.
- Yo-yo dieting leads to a loss of lean tissue and an increased risk of heart disease. However, it has no permanent effect on BMR.

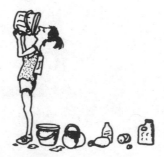

Gaining weight

There are two ways to gain weight: either by increasing your lean mass or by increasing your fat mass. Both will register as weight gain on the scales but result in a very different body composition and appearance!

Lean weight gain can be achieved by combining the right type of strength training programme with a balanced diet. Strength (resistance) training provides the stimulus for muscle growth while your diet provides the right amount of energy (calories) and nutrients to enable your muscles to grow at the optimal rate. One without the other will result in minimal lean weight gain.

What type of training is best for gaining weight?

Resistance training (weight training) is the best way to stimulate muscle growth. Research shows that the fastest gains in size and strength are achieved using relatively heavy weights that can be lifted strictly for 6–10 repetitions per set. If you can do more than 10–12 repetitions at a particular weight, your size gains will be less, but you may still achieve improvements in muscular endurance, strength and power.

Concentrate on the 'compound' exercises, such as bench press, squat, shoulder press and lat pull-down, as these work the largest muscle groups of the body together with neighbouring muscles that act as 'assistors' or 'synergists'. These type of exercises stimulate the largest number of muscle fibres in one movement and are therefore the most effective and quickest way to gain muscle mass. Keep the smaller isolation exercises, such as biceps concentration curls or tricep kickbacks, to a minimum; these produce slower mass gains and should only be added to your workout occasionally for variety.

Training for muscle gain

Certain compound exercises, such as dead lifts, clean and jerks, snatches and squats, not only stimulate the 'prime mover' muscles, but also have a powerful anabolic ('systemic') effect on the whole body and the central nervous system. These are the classic mass builders and should be included once a week in any serious muscle/strength training programme.

To stimulate the maximal number of muscle fibres in a muscle group, select one to three basic exercises and aim to do 4–12 total sets for that muscle group. Latest research suggests that doing fewer sets (4–8) but using heavier weights (80–90% of your one-rep maximum ie. the maximum weight which can be lifted through one complete repetition) results in faster size and strength gains. If you exercise that muscle group to exhaustion, you will need to allow up to seven days for recuperation before repeating the same workout. So, aim to train each muscle group once a week (on average). In practice, divide your body parts (e.g. chest, legs, shoulders, back, arms) into three or four, and train one part per workout.

Always use strict training form and, ideally, have a partner to 'spot' for you so that you can use near-maximal weights safely. Always remember to warm up each muscle group beforehand with light aerobic training (e.g. exercise bike) and some relevant stretches. Ensure you also stretch the muscles after (and, ideally, in between each part of) the workout to help relieve soreness.

How much weight can I expect to gain?

How much lean weight you can expect to gain depends on three main factors:

◆ genetics
◆ body type
◆ hormonal balance.

Your genetics determine the proportion of different types of fibres in your muscles. The fast twitch (type II) fibres generate power and increase in size more readily than the slow twitch (type I or endurance) fibres. So, if you naturally have plenty of fast twitch fibres in your muscles, you will probably respond faster to a strength training programme than someone who has a higher proportion of slow twitch fibres. Unfortunately, you cannot convert slow twitch into fast twitch fibres – hence two people can follow exactly the same training programme, yet the one with lots of fast twitch muscle fibres will naturally gain weight faster than the other.

Your natural body type also affects how fast you gain lean weight. An ectomorph (naturally slim build with long lean limbs, narrow shoulders and hips) will find it harder to gain weight than a mesomorph (muscular, athletic build with wide shoulders and narrow hips) who tends to gain muscle readily. An endomorph (stocky, rounded build with wide shoulders and hips and an even distribution of fat) gains both fat and muscle readily.

People with a higher natural level of the male (anabolic) sex hormones, such as testosterone, will also gain muscle faster. That is why women cannot achieve the muscle mass or size of men unless they take anabolic steroids.

However, no matter what your genetics, natural build and hormonal balance, everyone can gain muscle and improve their shape with strength training. It is just that it takes some people longer than others.

How fast can I expect to gain weight?

Muscle and strength gains are usually faster at the start of a strength programme. Gains are often periodic as each improvement is interspersed with a plateau. As with a weight loss programme, aim to gain weight gradually. After an initial, relatively fast gain, expect to gain no more than 1–2 lb (0.5–1 kg) per month or 0.25–1% of your body weight per week. Monitor your body composition rather than simply your weight. If you gain weight much more than 2 lb per month on an established programme, then you are likely to be gaining fat!

How much should I eat?

To gain weight and muscle strength at the optimal rate you need to be in a slight positive energy balance, i.e. consuming slightly more calories than you need for maintenance. Estimate your current calorie intake by keeping a food diary for a few consecutive days. Since it takes 2500 extra calories to gain 1 lb muscle, you need to increase your food intake. In practice, slow gainers should add an extra 500 kcal to their daily diet; fast gainers may need less (300–500 kcal). Not all of these extra calories are converted into muscle – some will be used for digestion and absorption, given off as heat or used for physical activity.

Do I need to eat extra protein?

Contrary to popular belief, extra protein is not automatically converted into muscle! Although strength training increases your protein requirements (*see* Chapter 3), these should be easily satisfied by a balanced diet, if you are eating enough food generally. Protein intake is normally proportional to calorie intake – the more food you eat, the more protein you obtain, as it is found in a wide range of foods. Aim to consume daily between 1.4 and 1.7 g per kg body weight when following a strength training programme.

How often should I eat?

Eating at frequent and regular intervals ensures a steady supply of nutrients to your recuperating muscles. Start refuelling your glycogen stores as soon as possible after training – a minimum of 50 g carbohydrate every two hours is recommended (*see* Chapter 2). Protein breakdown (catabolism) is highest straight after training, so you should leave at least 2–4 hours before consuming high protein foods. This is when the rate of building (anabolism) begins to exceed the rate of breakdown.
In practice, divide your daily intake into at least five or six meals and snacks, and avoid leaving gaps longer than 3–4 hours.

Eating tips for hard gainers

- Increase your calorie intake by approximately 500 kcal/day.
- Aim for a gradual weight gain – 1–2 lb per month.
- Eat at least 5–6 meals and snacks a day (every 2–3 hours).
- If you cannot eat large meals, include more snacks between meals.
- Include a mixture of high and low fibre foods in your diet so it is not too bulky and filling, e.g. wholemeal and white bread, fresh fruit and fruit juice.
- Obtain your extra calories from low bulk, nutritious foods, e.g. dried fruit, milk-based drinks, yoghurt, fruit juice, energy bars or nuts, rather than filling up on high calorie or fatty foods, e.g. biscuits, chocolate or cakes, which are low in essential nutrients.

SUMMARY OF KEY POINTS

- Gaining weight involves a combination of strength training and a balanced diet.
- The rate of weight gain depends on genetics, body type and hormonal balance. On average, a lean weight gain of 0.5–1 kg per month is recommended.
- To gain muscle strength and size, a slight positive energy balance is needed, and a protein intake of between 1.4–1.7 g/kg body weight is recommended.

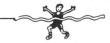

10

Disordered eating

In the general population in the UK it is estimated there are 125,000 bulimics and 70,000 anorexics (of which one in 10 cases are men). These figures may well represent only the tip of the iceberg, since many cases are not reported. However, there is now increasing evidence that the incidence of eating disorders is even higher among sportspeople, to the extent that a newly defined category called 'disordered eating', 'sub-clinical eating disorder', or 'anorexia athletica' has been defined by researchers. This chapter examines the possible reasons why athletes develop disordered eating patterns, and identifies the warning signs and symptoms. It also gives suggestions on how to approach someone suspected of having a disorder.

How common are eating disorders among sportspeople?

Eating disorders are more common among sportswomen than men, with US studies suggesting that up to 62% have some form of disordered eating. Surveys of élite female runners have found that many are obsessed with calorie counting and follow restricted, imbalanced diets: a recent survey of more than 4000 recreational runners found that 24% of the women, as opposed to 8% of the men, had attitudes to food suggestive of a major eating disorder. A study at Wolverhampton University found that two thirds of ballet dancers were underweight with a Body Mass Index (BMI) below 20 (the normal range is 20–25). One in three had a BMI less than 18.

About 0.2% of the male population is reported to suffer from anorexia nervosa, although the true figure is likely to be much higher, since men are much less likely to seek medical help, tending to see eating disorders as a woman's problem. In general, though, sportsmen are less likely than women to develop an eating disorder, partly because they experience less pressure to conform to a certain body shape and partly because they have a higher lean body weight and lower body fat than women anyway. They usually have less need or desire to lose or control their weight, and are less likely to experience negative feelings about their weight or shape. They are more likely to use exercise than dieting or purging as a means of weight control.

Sports considered most 'at risk' for men include weight category sports, such as wrestling and boxing; aesthetic sports, such as bodybuilding; and those where weight affects performance, such as jockeying or long distance running.

Why are sportspeople more prone to eating disorders?

Studies have found that, compared to the general population, many sportspeople show a higher level of body dissatisfaction, a greater pre-occupation with weight and body shape, and more disordered patterns of eating. One of the problems is that emphasis is placed on body weight and aesthetic qualities rather than on health, fitness and performance. Thus, those athletes in sports requiring a thin or very lean physique, either for performance or aesthetic reasons, tend to have a more distorted body image and are, therefore, at higher risk of developing an eating disorder.

Researchers have identified certain personality characteristics in individuals at risk of developing an eating disorder. These include obsession, competitiveness, perfectionism, compulsiveness and a high degree of self motivation – characteristics required for top level sports performance. So it is possible that some people with a predisposition to eating disorders are attracted to certain sports. In this situation, the sport can become a camouflage for the illness, as it is easy for the individual to hide behind its requirement for thinness. Some people may also be attracted to the training demands of a particular sport, using it as a method to control their weight.

Can sport cause an eating disorder?

A number of researchers have suggested that strenuous exercise regimes and restrictive diets can initiate eating disorders. Hard training, they say, can suppress appetite, which decreases food intake and body weight, and consequently increases the desire to exercise harder, thus creating a vicious circle. Also, in certain sports, athletes may be put under greater pressure to lose weight or conform to a certain body shape, which can precipitate an eating disorder. In one survey of gymnasts, where 67% had been told by their coaches that they were too heavy, 75% did, in fact, use pathogenic methods (e.g. starving, laxative abuse, excessive training) to control their weight.

Can sport cause eating disorders in predisposed athletes?

Clearly, not all athletes who participate in a thinness-demand sport or embark on a diet go on to develop an eating disorder, therefore a degree of susceptibility must be present at the start. It is more likely, then, that certain sports or exercise programmes precipitate rather than cause an eating disorder in one already at risk (e.g. with an existing history of family conflicts, low self esteem, confused social role).

Sport and exercise give the 'predisposed' athlete a sense of achievement and control over her body. The training involved provides another means by which to lose weight or body fat, and the positive relationship between leanness and sports performance further legitimises the athlete's pursuit of thinness. Thus, the fitness programme or sport reinforces the eating disorder 'personality' while at the same time acting as a socially acceptable camouflage for the disorder.

What is disordered eating?

The pressure to be thin or lean causes many athletes to restrict their calorie intake in order to attain an unnatural body shape. This is not simply to improve their performance but more for aesthetic reasons. A number of top international sportswomen admit to a greater concern about their appearance than is merited by their performance in competition.

Table 1: *Disordered eating – 'at risk' sports*

Endurance	Long distance running Long distance cycling
Aesthetic	Gymnastics Figure skating Ballet Competitive aerobics Bodybuilding Synchronised swimming
Weight category	Lightweight rowing Boxing Wrestling Judo/karate Weight lifting/powerlifting Bodybuilding

Disordered eating is not a clinical eating disorder as it does not meet the American Psychiatric Association's (APA) official criteria for anorexia nervosa or bulimia nervosa, although it includes some, but not all, of the major symptoms.

What are the symptoms of disordered eating?

Sufferers have an intense fear of gaining weight or becoming fat, even though their weight is normal or below normal. They are totally preoccupied with food and calories, and their weight and body shape. They also tend to have a distorted body image; thinking they are fat when they are not. They attempt to lose weight by strict dieting, usually consuming below 1200 kcal a day, and exercise excessively. They have chaotic eating patterns and often irregular or absent periods. Bingeing and purging (e.g. laxative and diuretic use) are common, although the actual amount eaten during a 'binge' is not that much greater than a normal sized meal.

What are the health consequences of disordered eating?

The strict dieting characteristic of disordered eating leads to low energy levels. Combined with excessive exercise, extreme fatigue can result. This, along with a reduced aerobic capacity and cardio-vascular changes, can reduce performance ability. Recovery from injury will be poor and slower, and susceptibility to infection increased. The chaotic and restricted eating patterns can also lead to electrolyte imbalances and menstrual irregularities, sometimes even to amenorrhoea. With a reduced calcium intake, bone loss and premature osteoporosis become a real risk. Finally, the sufferer may experience depression.

Table 2: Anorexia nervosa

Characteristics	Warning signs	Health consequences
◆ severe weight loss ◆ self induced starvation ◆ obsessive fear of weight gain ◆ low self esteem ◆ fear of fatness ◆ distorted body image ◆ depression and anxiety ◆ perfectionism ◆ obsessiveness ◆ high need for approval ◆ social withdrawal ◆ obsessive exercise	◆ extreme thinness and weight loss ◆ excessive facial and body hair ◆ claiming to be fat when thin ◆ eating very little ◆ great interest in food and calories ◆ anxiety and arguments about food ◆ amenorrhoea ◆ feeling cold/bluish extremities ◆ restlessness/ sleeping very little ◆ obsessive weighing	◆ reduced physical performance ◆ decreased aerobic capacity ◆ increased susceptibility to infection ◆ slow recovery from injury ◆ electrolyte imbalances ◆ amenorrhoea ◆ cardiac arrhythmias ◆ increased risk of bone loss and early osteoporosis ◆ hypotension ◆ hypothermia ◆ gastrointestinal problems

Table 3: Bulimia nervosa

Characteristics	Warning signs	Health consequences
◆ bingeing on large amounts of food (up to 5000 kcal)	◆ tooth decay/ enamel erosion	◆ menstrual irregularities
◆ guilt and remorse after bingeing	◆ puffy face	◆ enamel erosion and gum disease
◆ purging – vomiting or laxative abuse	◆ normal weight or weight fluctuations	◆ gastrointestinal problems
◆ starvation	◆ frequent weighing	◆ bowel problems
◆ low self esteem	◆ disappearing after meals to get rid of food	◆ dehydration
◆ impulsiveness	◆ secretive eating	◆ electrolyte imbalances
◆ depression, anger, anxiety	◆ menstrual disturbances	◆ cardiovascular complications
◆ body dissatisfaction and image distortion		◆ hypotension
◆ high need for approval		
◆ excessive exercise		
◆ obsession with food and weight		

How can athletes with an eating disorder continue training?

It seems extraordinary that athletes with apparently very low calorie intakes continue to exercise and compete to the same degree. Undoubtedly a combination of psychological and physiological factors are involved. Psychologically, anorexics are able to push themselves to exercise despite feelings of exhaustion as sufferers are typically strong willed and highly motivated to succeed. On the physiological side, it has been suggested that the body adapts to the high training demands but low calorie intake by becoming more energy efficient, reducing its metabolic rate (sometimes by 10–30%).

To overcome physical and emotional fatigue, many anorexics and bulimics use stimulants, such as caffeinated drinks (e.g. strong coffee, 'diet' cola), for energy. However, in the long term, performance will fall.

As glycogen and nutrient stores become chronically depleted the athlete's health will suffer and optimal performance can no longer be sustained. Maximal oxygen consumption decreases, chronic fatigue sets in and the athlete becomes more susceptible to injury and infection. Optimal performance cannot, therefore, be sustained indefinitely.

Some scientists believe that some athletes under-report their food intake and, in fact, eat more than they admit. For example, a study at Indiana University on nine highly trained cross-country runners found that they were eating, on average, 2100 kcal per day, though their predicted energy expenditure was 300 kcal. After analysing the results of their Food Attitude Questionnaire, the researchers suggested that many had a poor body image and had inaccurately reported what they ate during the study.

How should I approach someone suspected of having an eating disorder?

This requires great tact and sensitivity. Sufferers are likely to deny that they have a problem; they may feel embarrassed and their self esteem threatened. It is vital, therefore, to avoid direct confrontation about eating behaviour or physical symptoms. Tread very gently – do not suddenly present 'evidence', and avoid accusations.

Once the sufferer admits to having an eating problem, suggest that it would be best to have an initial consultation with an eating disorders specialist. Various forms of professional help are available, from trained counsellors in self-help organisations to private eating disorders clinics (*see* pages 173–74), or a GP may refer them for treatment within a multidisciplinary team of psychologists and dietitians.

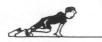

Table 4: *Have you got an eating problem?*

This questionnaire is not intended as a diagnostic method for eating problems nor as a substitute for a full diagnosis by an eating disorders specialist.
◆ Do you exercise specifically to lose weight or fat? ◆ Do you worry about or dislike your body shape? ◆ Do you often 'feel fat' one day and 'thin' the next? ◆ Do your friends/family insist that you are slim while you feel fat? ◆ Do you feel guilty after eating a high calorie or high fat meal? ◆ Do you constantly scrutinise food labels to check the nutritional content? ◆ Do you avoid certain foods even though you want to eat them? ◆ Do you feel stressed or guilty if your normal diet or exercise routine is interrupted? ◆ Do you often decline invitations to meals and social occasions involving food in case you might have to eat something fattening?

Table 5: *Learning to break the habit*

This guide is not intended as a treatment for an eating disorder. Treatment should always be sought from an eating disorders specialist.
◆ Learn to accept and like your body's shape – emphasise your good points. ◆ Realise that reducing your body fat will not solve deep rooted problems or an emotional crisis. ◆ Don't set rigid eating rules for yourself and feel guilty when you break them. ◆ Don't ban or feel guilty about eating any foods. ◆ Establish a sensible healthy eating pattern rather than a strict diet. ◆ Listen to your natural appetite cues – learn to eat when you are hungry. ◆ If you do overeat, don't try to 'pay for it' later by starving yourself. ◆ Enjoy your exercise or sport for its own sake: have fun instead of enduring torture to lose body fat.

Useful organisations

Eating Disorders Association, Sackville Place, 44–48 Magdalen Street, Norfolk NR3 1JU. Tel: 01603 621414

National Centre for Eating Disorders, 54 New Road, Esher, Surrey. Tel: 01372 469493

Maisner Centre for Eating Disorders, PO Box 464, Hove, East Sussex BN3 2BN. Tel: 01273 729818

British Association for Counselling, 1 Regent Place, Rugby, Warwickshire CV21 2PJ. Tel: 01788 578328

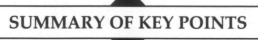

SUMMARY OF KEY POINTS

- Disordered eating patterns are increasingly common among athletes and fitness participants; it is estimated that up to 62% of female athletes may be affected.
- Disordered eating, characterised by a preoccupation with food, food restriction and a poor body image, is regarded as a sub-clinical eating disorder as it includes some but not all the criteria for defining a clinical eating disorder such as anorexia nervosa and bulimia nervosa.
- Athletes share many of the same personality characteristics as people with clinical eating disorders: obsessiveness, compulsiveness, competitiveness, perfectionism.
- Sports most 'at risk' include endurance sports (leanness is believed to be an advantage for performance), aesthetic sports (leanness is believed to be an important judging criteria in competition), and weight category sports.
- Many sportspeople appear to have a distorted body image and a higher level of body dissatisfaction than the general population.
- There is no single cause of clinical or sub-clinical eating disorders. It is likely that certain sports may precipitate an eating disorder in predisposed people, rather than be the cause of the eating disorder.
- The health consequences of disordered eating include chronic fatigue, a reduction in performance, susceptibility to infection and injury, menstrual irregularities, amenorrhoea, increased risk of stress fractures and osteoporosis.
- Sufferers should be approached with tact and sensitivity, then guided towards professional help by an eating disorders specialist or counsellor.

11

Putting it all into practice

Now that you have a good understanding of the main principles of sports nutrition, the time has come to put it all into practice. Knowing the theory is only half the battle. Being able to fit it in with your lifestyle is the other half.

This chapter addresses some of the most common problems faced by athletes and those leading an active lifestyle: eating on the run, in a hurry, on a budget, and adapting family meals. If you lead a busy lifestyle, it may be tempting to skip meals or rely on snacks that are high in fat or sugar. This chapter gives you plenty of practical ideas for healthy snacks that you can take with you. It also provides useful suggestions on overcoming the difficulties of putting theory into practice.

As more athletes are giving up meat and choosing a vegetarian diet, this chapter explains how you can get all the nutrients needed for good performance on a meat-free diet. It also highlights the special dietary problems faced by female athletes, and suggests how to avoid them. Finally the chapter gives comprehensive yet simple advice to competitive sportspeople on what to eat before, during and after competitions.

I often have to eat on the run. What can I do?

Try to organise your food in advance. If you don't have time for proper meals, take a supply of healthy snacks with you. This way you can keep up your energy levels, refuel after training and ensure you are getting a good intake of nutrients. Plan to eat a small snack every two or three hours – *see* Table 1 for ideas on high carbohydrate, low fat, portable foods.

If you have to buy takeaways and ready made snacks, choose sandwiches with low fat fillings, jacket potatoes (with baked beans/cottage cheese/chicken/fish), pizza slices (with vegetable based topping), pasta and rice salads.

Always make time to relax while eating. If you are rushed or tense, you may develop indigestion, heartburn and trapped air, all of which can be very uncomfortable, especially if you will be training later on! So, reserve at least 5–10 minutes to sit down, unwind and eat slowly.

Never skip meals altogether or leave long gaps without food. This will result in low blood sugar levels, poor glycogen replenishment, a lower nutrient intake and greater lethargy. So, the key is to be prepared and plan your eating around your daily schedule.

Table 1: *Snacks for eating on the run*

> ◆ Sandwiches/rolls/pitta/bagels (filled with cottage cheese/peanut butter/banana/salad/honey/marmite/tuna/chicken/turkey/ham)
> ◆ Low fat yoghurt and fromage frais
> ◆ Fresh fruit (e.g. apples, bananas, nectarines, grapes)
> ◆ English muffins/scones/crumpets/potato cakes
> ◆ Scotch pancakes
> ◆ Dried fruit and cereal bars
> ◆ Fruit juice or cordial (diluted)
> ◆ Nuts and dried fruit mixtures
> ◆ Rice cakes/crackers/breakfast cereal

How can I eat cheaply but healthily?

A healthy diet need not be expensive if you make just a few simple changes to your shopping and eating habits. In fact, many of the most nutritious foods are inexpensive and readily available: potatoes, pasta, oats, rice and other cereal grains (e.g. bulgar wheat, couscous, millet), pulses (dried or tinned) and milk. These foods can be used to form the basis of your diet, for example: jacket potatoes with fillings; pasta, rice and grain dishes with a simple sauce; grain based salads; curries, salads, stews and soups based on pulses and vegetables in season; milk drinks and puddings (e.g. custard, rice pudding).

◆ Buy fruit and vegetables in season; look out for special offers in the shops or buy from market stalls, if possible.

- Avoid ready prepared meals and 'convenience' products – they may seem to save you time, but its cheaper and just as easy to make large amounts of the same dish yourself and freeze the remainder.
- High protein foods from plants (pulses, cereals, nuts, soya products) are less expensive than those from animals (meat, poultry, fish, eggs), so make greater use of these in your diet, e.g. risotto with beans instead of chicken.
- If you feel hungry, fill up on inexpensive, nutritious foods like bread, toast and fruit instead of other less nutritious snacks, such as confectionery bars, crisps and cakes.
- Buy the largest packs of breakfast cereals, frozen fish and poultry, pasta, rice, and dairy products as these are usually cheaper. Organise your storage space well or share the pack with a friend!

I don't have much time to cook and prepare healthy meals. What can I do?

Healthy meals can be very quick and easy to prepare. Many require no or very little cooking. Here are a few tips:

- Make larger quantities than you need of soups, casseroles, potatoes, pasta, rice, etc., then cover and keep the remainder in the fridge or freezer. Before eating, add extra ingredients (e.g. beans, poultry, vegetables or sauce) as toppings or fillings.
- Make a large bowl of vegetables or fruit salad, enough to last 2–3 days, and keep in the fridge so you have an instant supply.
- The following speedy meals can be made in less than 10 minutes: baked beans or spaghetti on toast: pizza made with ready made base, tinned tomatoes and cheese; sandwiches and pitta; pasta with tomato/vegetable sauce; eggs or cheese on toast; baked potato with beans/cheese/tuna.

In fact, there's no need even to cook! Make substantial sandwiches using the ideas in the Sandwich box (Table 2).

I often have to eat late in the evening. What are my best choices?

If you train in the evening and do not arrive home until late, you should plan to have most of your food during the morning and

177

Table 2: *Sandwich box*

Bread
Cut thick slices from any of the following breads:
Multi grain, rye, sourdough, herb, Italian bread with olives, sun dried tomatoes or onions, Spanish bread with sunflower seeds, baguettes, ciabatta, country style bread

Fillings
Any combination of the following:
- Low fat soft cheese, dates and walnuts
- Hummous, lettuce and onion slices
- Peanut butter and banana
- Turkey and cranberry sauce
- Cottage cheese and dried/fresh apricots
- Salmon, watercress and low calorie dressing
- Ham, pears and lettuce
- Sun dried tomatoes, mozzarella and green salad leaves
- Tuna, red kidney beans and tabasco
- Chopped chicken, sweetcorn, onion and fromage frais
- Reduced fat hard cheese and pineapple
- Egg, lettuce, red pepper and low calorie salad dressing
- Grated carrot, raisins and cashews

afternoon. Have a substantial breakfast and make lunch your main meal of the day. Include frequent high carbohydrate snacks in between, with a snack about 1–2 hours before your evening training sessions. That way you will feel less hungry before and after training.

It is still important to eat after training to refuel your glycogen stores, but avoid a large or fatty meal which takes a long time to digest. Good late evening choices include pasta with a tomato based sauce, breakfast cereal, fruit and milk, beans on toast and thick sandwiches. Try to leave at least one or two hours before retiring to bed, as a full stomach can make you feel uncomfortable and disrupt your sleep.

I have to eat the same meals as the rest of my family!

The whole family can benefit from eating healthy meals – there is no need to prepare separate dishes. Simply fill up on larger portions of high carbohydrate foods, such as bread, pasta and potatoes, avoid large helpings of rich sauces and trim off any fat from meat.

Most traditional family meals can be easily adapted to contain less fat and more carbohydrate without affecting the taste or enjoyment. For example:

- Substitute low fat milk for full fat milk in sauces, custard and puddings.
- Sauté onions or meat in minimal amounts of oil.
- Omit the butter or oil in sauces and thicken with cornflour.
- Add extra vegetables or pulses to stews, bolognese, soups or curries.
- Reduce the amount of fat in puddings, cakes and desserts and serve with extra fruit or yoghurt.

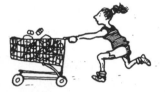

I like eating out. What are the best choices from the menu?

You can still enjoy eating out and eating healthily provided you make the right menu choices. Check below.

Table 3: Restaurant guide

	Good choices	**Unhealthy choices**
Pizzeria	Tomato, vegetable, ham, spicy chicken, or seafood pizza toppings	Salami, mince, beef, pepperoni, extra cheese toppings
Hamburger joint	Plain, grilled hamburger, flame grilled chicken	Large burgers, fries, doughnuts, apple pies
Steak house	Grilled steak, salads, jacket potatoes, fruit	Fried/battered fish, garlic mushrooms, garlic bread, scampi, steak with creamy sauces, puddings

	Good choices	Unhealthy choices
Indian	Chicken tikka, tandoori chicken, dahl, channa dahl, rice, naan bread, chappati, dry vegetable curries	Meat curries, meat dansak/korma/ madras, samosa, bhajis, puri, paratha
Chinese	Chicken, vegetable or prawn chop suey, stir fried vegetables, seafood or chicken, rice, noodles	Duck dishes, sweet and sour pork balls, fried noodles
French	Grilled fish, meat (e.g. steak au poivre), boeuf bourguignonne, poultry dishes without creamy sauces, ratatouille, salads (e.g. niçoise), bouillabaisse (fish stew), vegetables, consommé, sorbet	Cream or butter sauces (e.g. à la normandie, béarnaise), buttered vegetables, pastry dishes, profiteroles
Greek	Greek salad, tomato or cucumber salad, tzatzika, hoummous, pitta, dolmadhes, stuffed tomatoes, souvlakia, grilled or barbecued fish, fresh fruit, Greek yoghurt	Taramasalata, moussaka, lamb dishes, pastitsio, keftethakia (meatballs), spicy sausages, baklava
Spanish/Portugese	Paella, grilled fish, shellfish dishes, salads, gazpacho, tortillas	Buttery/oily sauces, fried fish pies, fried chicken
Japanese	Sushi, sashmi, sukiyaki, teryaki chicken	Tempura dishes

	Good choices	Unhealthy choices
Mexican	Bean burrito, tortillas or tostadas with beans/vegetable chilli, fajitas with vegetables/chicken, guacamole	Tortilla chips, potato skins, beef chilli, tortillas/burritos with beef, chimichangas
Thai	Steamed fish, rice and vegetable dishes, seafood salad	Prawn crackers, fried noodles or rice
Italian	Grissini, ciabatta, pasta with tomato/vegetable or seafood sauces (e.g. neopolitan, primavera, spinach), risotto, gnocchi, grilled chicken/fish, pasta filled with spinach/ricotta	Pasta with creamy/buttery/meat based sauce (e.g. carbonara, alfredo, bolognese), lasagne, cannelloni

Can a vegetarian diet provide all the nutrients I need?

A well planned vegetarian diet that excludes meat and fish can provide all the energy and nutrients needed by athletes and fitness participants. The nutrients which receive most concern are listed in Table 4, together with their non-meat sources and relevant advice.

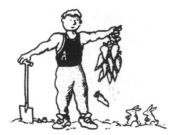

Table 4: *Planning a well balanced, vegetarian diet*

Nutrient	Sources	Advice
Protein	Milk, cheese, yoghurt, eggs, beans, lentils, peas, nuts, seeds, soya products (e.g. soya 'milk', TVP, tofu, tempeh), quorn	Eating a mixture of plant protein foods over the day will ensure an adequate intake of all essential amino acids (protein complementation). Choose lower fat versions of dairy products to reduce fat intake
Iron	Wholemeal bread, whole grains, nuts, pulses, green vegetables (e.g. broccoli, watercress), fortified soya products, fortified breakfast cereals, seeds, dried fruit	Eating vitamin C rich foods (e.g. fruit, vegetables, fruit juice) at the same time as iron rich foods greatly improves iron absorption
Vitamin B12	Dairy products, eggs, fortified foods (e.g. soya products, breakfast cereals, yeast extract)	As vitamin B12 is found naturally only in animal products, vegans should include B12-fortified products in their diet or take a supplement
Calcium	Dairy products, sunflower and sesame seeds, spinach, broccoli, almonds, brazil nuts, fortified soya products (e.g. tofu), figs	Vegan diets are often low in calcium so more careful planning is required

Nutrient	Sources	Advice
Zinc	Whole grains, wholemeal bread, pulses, nuts, seeds, eggs	Avoid bran and bran enriched foods as fibre can bind zinc and reduce its absorption

Are vegetarians healthier than meat-eaters?

Scientific studies of vegetarians have found that they have a longer lifespan, mainly due to their lower rate of heart disease. The longer the duration of vegetarianism, the lower the risk. The consensus is that vegetarian diets seem to offer a number of major health benefits. The 12 year Oxford Health Study (1994) of more than 6000 vegetarians and 5000 meat-eaters found that vegetarians have 30% less risk of heart disease, 40% less risk of cancer (especially breast and colon), and a significantly lower risk of bowel disorders, diabetes and osteoporosis. Compared with meat-eaters, vegetarians have lower blood pressure and lower blood cholesterol, and are typically leaner. One study found that only 5.4% of vegetarians were obese compared with 19.4% in a group of non vegetarians. This is probably due to their lower fat intakes.

Some of the benefits of a vegetarian diet may be due to a healthier lifestyle (e.g. not smoking, taking more exercise), but researchers believe that it could also be due to a higher intake of antioxidants, especially from fruit and vegetables, and of dietary fibre, or a lower intake of saturated fat. It is probably due to a combination of these factors.

Can a vegetarian diet support a hard training programme?

Increasing numbers of athletes are giving up meat, and there are many well known names who have converted to vegetarianism. Researchers in Germany recently compared the nutritional intakes of vegetarian and non vegetarian endurance runners. They found that energy, carbohydrate, fat and protein intakes were similar. However, the vegetarians ate more fibre, polyunsaturated fatty acids and less saturated fatty acids and cholesterol. They also achieved higher intakes of almost all vitamins and minerals, and exceeded the recommended intakes. Interestingly, they had higher intakes of iron due to the inclusion of plenty of pulses, green vegetables and whole grains. Other studies have found that vegetarian diets do not adversely affect aerobic or anaerobic capacity and that vegetarian athletes are therefore at no disadvantage.

Are there any drawbacks with a vegetarian diet?

As with any dietary change, it is important to plan your diet well and gain as much knowledge about vegetarian nutrition as possible. Some athletes (mainly women) adopt a vegetarian or vegan diet in order to lose weight or in the misguided belief that it will solve other problems. It thereby serves as a camouflage for disordered eating. Often in this scenario the athlete fails to substitute suitable foods in place of meat or to consume enough nutrients to support training.

A very bulky vegetarian diet that includes lots of high fibre foods may be too filling for athletes with high energy needs. This means they may not be able to eat enough calories, in which case you should include more compact sources of carbohydrate (e.g. dried fruit, fruit juice) and include a mixture of both whole grain and refined grain products (e.g. wholemeal and white bread) in your diet.

Do female athletes have special needs?

In general, female athletes have lower intakes of calcium, iron, riboflavin and folic acid compared with males, and this may adversely affect their health and performance. This difference is mainly due to a lower food intake generally – females are more likely to be dieting or restricting their food in order to lose or avoid gaining weight.

Calcium

Calcium is important for bone health. A low intake of calcium together with intense training, low body fat levels, amenorrhoea and a low calorie intake can increase the risk of stress fractures and osteoporosis. Indeed, women involved in low body weight sports, such as endurance running and gymnastics, have a higher rate of amenorrhoea, which is associated with reduced levels of oestrogen. This in turn leads to increased bone mineral loss. Researchers have found that amenorrhoeic female athletes have a lower bone density than athletes with normal periods. This puts them at risk of developing early osteoporosis. In one study, researchers found significantly lower measures of bone density in the spines of runners who had absent or irregular periods compared with normally menstruating runners. Fortunately, it has also been found that when athletes begin to have normal periods again, their bone density increases.

Current research suggests that an adequate calcium intake may help to offset calcium loss from the bones. Therefore, it is important that all female athletes consume at least the RNI for calcium (700 mg). Indeed, a number of scientists recommend that amenorrhoeic athletes consume double this amount (1200–1500 mg). Good sources of calcium include milk and dairy products, tinned fish with soft edible bones (e.g. sardines), pulses, dark green leafy vegetables, figs, shellfish, fortified white bread and flour, nuts and seeds.

Iron

Iron deficiency anaemia is more common among female athletes than males. A large proportion of women have low iron stores, which itself may not be an immediate problem, but it can easily develop into iron deficiency anaemia if iron needs increase (e.g. during pregnancy) or if losses increase (e.g. heavy menstrual periods). Heavy training can also lead to increased iron losses, thus exacerbating the problem. The early symptoms of anaemia, such as fatigue, headaches, light headedness and breathlessness, often go unnoticed and may be put down to other causes. If symptoms persist and you feel excessively tired despite plenty of rest, you should consult your doctor for a proper diagnosis.

Many female athletes avoid red meat (the most readily absorbed form of iron) or eat only very small amounts, so it is important to get iron from other foods, such as pulses, wholegrain cereals, fortified breakfast cereals, dark green vegetables, dried fruit and eggs. Low calorie intakes (less than 1500 kcal) usually mean low iron intakes too, so make sure that you include plenty of the above foods if you are on a weight loss programme. Remember, vitamin C rich foods enhance iron absorption, so include fruit and vegetables at the same time.

Iron supplements are not normally routinely advised for female athletes because they can have side effects (e.g. constipation) and may lead to mineral imbalances. If you suspect you are at risk of anaemia, consult your doctor for a diagnosis. He will then advise you whether you need to take supplements.

Riboflavin

Exercise increases the requirements for most of the B vitamins, including riboflavin. Female athletes who restrict their food intake tend to have low riboflavin intakes since this is proportional to calorie intake. Make sure you include plenty of riboflavin-rich foods in your diet, such as low fat milk and dairy products, eggs and chicken.

Folic acid

Women generally tend to have a low intake of folic acid, one of the B vitamins involved in cell division and red blood cell formation. It is particularly important during the first 12 weeks of pregnancy, since a deficiency increases the risk of neural tube defects such as spina bifida. The Department of Health advise a supplement containing 0.4 mg folic acid for all women planning a pregnancy, to be taken until the 12th week after conception. However, latest research suggests that other nutrients, such as vitamin B12, may also be important, so aim to eat a nutritious diet that includes good amounts of all the B vitamins.

What should I eat in the week before a competition?

During the week before a competition, aim to fill your glycogen stores so that you enter with a full fuel supply. If you were entering a long distance car race, you would make sure that your petrol tank was filled to the brim with the best quality fuel before you started. That would give you the best possible chance of maintaining top speeds for longer. Therefore, give yourself the best advantage over your competitors by arriving at the competition with maximum glycogen stores. The best way to achieve this is to gradually taper your training and increase your carbohydrate intake during the final week.

Your total calorie intake should remain about the same as usual, but the balance of carbohydrate, fat and protein will change. Eat larger amounts of carbohydrate-rich foods (e.g. potatoes, bread, rice, dried fruit, carbohydrate drinks) and smaller amounts of fats and proteins. Aim to have a snack or meal every 2–3 hours. Ideally, your carbohydrate intake should be 60–70% of energy.

Is carbohydrate loading a good idea?

Carbohydrate loading is a technique originally devised in the 1960s to increase the muscles' glycogen stores above normal levels. This is advantageous in endurance events lasting two or more hours (e.g. long distance running or cycling) or for events that involve several heats or matches over a short period (e.g. tennis and rugby tournaments). It is unlikely to benefit you if your event lasts less than 90 minutes or if it involves short bursts of activity.

The original method involved three days of glycogen depletion (through exhaustive exercise and a low carbohydrate diet) followed by three days of glycogen loading (through reduced training and a high carbohydrate diet). However this method has a number of drawbacks. The depletion phase can leave you feeling excessively weak and drained, and you may not succeed in loading up sufficiently over the next three days. Latest research, however, has found that you can achieve equally good results by omitting the depletion phase, tapering training and gradually increasing your carbohydrate intake over 7 days. This can increase muscle glycogen stores by up to 30–40%.

Never try anything new before an important competition, so if you decide to try carbohydrate loading, rehearse it during training to find out what works best for you. You may need to try the technique more than once, adjusting the types and amounts of foods you eat. It is advisable not to carbohydrate load seriously more than 3–4 times a year.

When should I eat before my competition?

Plan to have your pre-competition meal 3–4 hours before the event. This will allow enough time for your stomach to empty sufficiently, and for blood sugar and insulin levels to normalise. Nervousness can slow down your digestion rate, so you may need to leave a little longer than usual between eating and competing.

Figure 1: *Carbohydrate loading*

Old technique

Depletion→→→→→→→→→→ Loading →→→→→→→→→→Competition

1	2	3	4	5	6	7

New technique

Taper training→→→→→→→→→ Rest →→→→→→→→→→→Competition

1	2	3	4	5	6	7

Increase carbohydrate intake→→→→→→→→→→→→→→→→→ Competition

What should I eat before my competition?

Your pre-competition meal should be:

- High in carbohydrate
- Low in fat
- Low in protein
- Low in fibre
- Not too bulky
- Enjoyable and familiar
- Easy to digest
- Accompanied by drink.

Suitable types of meals are given in the box on page 189. If you really do not feel like eating, have a liquid meal such as a carbohydrate drink, fruit juice, milkshake or a sports drink.

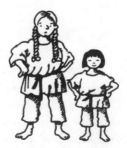

Table 5: Pre-competition meals

- ◆ Breakfast cereal with low fat milk
- ◆ Toast or bread with jam/honey
- ◆ Sandwiches or rolls with banana/honey/jam
- ◆ Pasta or rice with low fat sauce
- ◆ Buns, muffins
- ◆ Rice cakes or crackers with banana or jam
- ◆ Baked potato with low fat filling
- ◆ Fruit, e.g. bananas, oranges, grapes, raisins
- ◆ Energy bars
- ◆ Carbohydrate drinks

Should I eat or drink just before my competition?

Studies have shown that taking in a small amount (approximately 50 g) of carbohydrate (in solid or liquid form) just before exercise can help maintain blood sugar levels, delay fatigue and improve performance. The timing can range from 5 to 30 minutes, according to the individual, so experiment in training first! Provided you begin exercise soon afterwards, hypoglycaemia will be avoided because exercise suppresses insulin release.

You should also make sure that you are well hydrated before the competition (check the colour of your urine!), so aim to drink at least 300 ml of fluid about 30 minutes beforehand.

Choose foods or drinks with a high glycaemic index, such as a 300 ml carbohydrate drink (20% carbohydrate); a 500 ml isotonic sports drink; 2 large bananas with a glass of water; a confectionery bar with a glass of water.

Should I eat or drink during my competition?

If you are competing for more than 90 minutes, you may find that extra carbohydrate will help delay fatigue and maintain your performance, particularly in the latter stages. However, start to take this extra carbohydrate before fatigue sets in, after about 30 minutes, and carry on doing so at frequent intervals. Depending on your exercise intensity and duration, aim to take in 30–60 g carbohydrate/hour. If you are cycling, try taking foods such as energy bars, bananas, dried fruit bars or raisins with you (as well as drinks). If you are competing in matches and tournaments (e.g.

189

football, tennis), take suitable snacks and drinks for the intervals.

Any carbohydrate with a high glycaemic index makes a suitable snack, but you may find liquids easier to consume than solids. Isotonic sports drinks or carbohydrate (glucose polymer) drinks are usually helpful because they serve to replenish fluid losses and prevent dehydration as well as supplying carbohydrate. Avoid high fructose drinks as they are not absorbed as fast as sucrose, glucose and glucose polymers. They may also cause diarrhoea!

If you are competing for more than 90 minutes, avoid or delay dehydration by drinking 15–30 minutes before the start, thereafter every 15–20 minutes or whenever you have the chance. Drink as much as you feel comfortable with, ideally 150–300 ml.

Table 6: Recommended quantity of a 6% isotonic drink during exercise (60 g glucose/sucrose/glucose polymer dissolved in 1 litre water)

Moderate intensity (30 g carbohydrate/h)	Moderate – high intensity (45 g carbohydrate/h)	High intensity (60 g carbohydrate/h)
500 ml/h	750 ml/h	1000 ml/h

What should I eat between heats or after my competition?

If you compete in several heats, it's important to refuel and rehydrate as fast as possible so that you have a good chance of performing well in your next competition.

If you have only a few hours between heats, you may prefer liquid meals, such as sports drinks and carbohydrate drinks or protein/carbohydrate supplement drinks. These will help replace both glycogen and fluid. If you are able to eat solid food, choose carbohydrates with a high glycaemic index that you find easy to digest and not too filling. Try bananas, breakfast cereal, high carbohydrate bars (sports bars or fruit bars), oatmeal biscuits, dried fruit, home made muffins or rice cakes. Take these with you in your kit bag. Start eating and drinking as soon as possible after your heat.

If you have more than a few hours between heats or if you have finished competing, you will have time to eat a larger meal. Again, choose foods with a high glycaemic index to ensure rapid refuelling, but allow 3–4 hours between the meal and your next competition. Avoid rich or fatty meals (e.g. takeaway curries, chips, burgers) as these will delay refuelling and can make you feel bloated after competing. Don't forget to drink plenty of rehydrating fluid before embarking on that celebratory alcoholic drink!

SUMMARY OF KEY POINTS

◆ If you eat on the run, take a supply of healthy snacks with you to consume at regular intervals.

◆ If you need to eat on a budget, base your diet around basic nutritious foods such as cereals, pulses, starchy vegetables and milk. Buy fruit and vegetables in season and shop in bulk.

◆ If you have little time to prepare meals, cook larger quantities and save the remainder. Plan your weekly menu in advance and use some of the quick ideas given in this chapter.

◆ If you have to eat late at night, consume most of your food during the earlier part of the day, then have a moderate sized high carbohydrate snack/meal in the evening after training.

◆ If you eat out a lot, use the menu guide in this chapter to help you make the healthiest choices.

◆ A well planned vegetarian diet can provide all the nutrients needed by athletes for good health and performance. Vegans may need to use more fortified foods.

◆ Female athletes may be at greater risk of deficient intakes of iron, calcium, riboflavin and folic acid, due to their lower intakes of food generally.

◆ The pre-competition diet should be high in carbohydrate to ensure full glycogen stores, and include plenty of fluids to ensure you are well hydrated.

◆ The pre-competition meal should be taken 3–4 hours before-hand, be high in carbohydrate, low in fat and fibre, and easy to digest.

◆ Consuming an additional 50 g high GI carbohydrate immediately before competition may delay fatigue in events lasting more than 1 hour.

◆ Performance in events lasting > 90 min may be increased by consuming 30–60 g carbohydrate/hour in solid or liquid form.

12

The recipes

The following recipes are quick, simple and fun to make. They are specially designed for sportspeople who need to eat a diet high in carbohydrate, low in fat and rich in essential nutrients. Each recipe provides a nutritional analysis to help you put together numerous healthy menus.

The main meal recipes are divided into sections based on high carbohydrate foods to enable you to plan your meals according to the recommended nutritional guidelines. Recipes suitable for vegetarians contain no meat, poultry or fish and are marked with a 'V' symbol.

Rice and other grains

Rice is high in complex carbohydrates and makes a tasty and versatile base for main meals. Brown rice is a little higher in fibre and B vitamins than white, although it is not as high as other wholegrain cereals. Experiment with different types of rice: American, Italian, Basmati or wild. Try different types of grains, too: bulgar wheat, couscous, millet and barley. Most are available in supermarkets.

V

Beans 'n' Rice

This healthy combination appears in many American and West Indian cuisines. The beans can be black, red or white, and the dish can be spicy or mild – adapt it to taste.

Serves 2

1 tbsp (15 ml) oil
1 onion, chopped
1 green chilli, chopped finely
6 oz (175 g) rice
1 large tomato, chopped
¾ pint (450 ml) stock

15 oz (400 g) beans *or* cooked dried beans (e.g. red kidney beans, borlotti beans or black beans)
1 oz (25 g) creamed coconut
1 tbsp chopped coriander or parsley

- Heat oil in a pan.
- Add onion and cook for 5 minutes.
- Add chilli and rice and stir well for 2 minutes.
- Add tomato and stock.
- Bring to the boil, cover and simmer for 15 minutes.
- Add cooked beans and cook for a further 5 minutes.
- Gradually stir in creamed coconut until it has melted, followed by coriander or parsley.

Nutritional information (per serving):
Calories = 637; protein = 23 g; carbohydrate = 112 g; fat = 13.9 g; fibre = 12.8 g

Spicy Chicken with Rice

Serves 2

2 tsp (10 ml) sunflower oil
2 chicken breasts (approx. 6 oz (175 g) each)
6 oz (175 g) brown rice
1 onion, chopped

2 cloves garlic, crushed
1–2 tsp (5–10 ml) curry powder (to taste)
1 tbsp tomato purée
3 tbsp water

- Cook the chicken breasts under a hot grill for 10–15 minutes, turning a few times.
- Boil rice for 20–25 minutes.
- Meanwhile, heat oil in a large non-stick pan and cook onion for 5 minutes, until golden.
- Add garlic and curry powder and cook for a further 2 minutes.
- Cut chicken into chunks and add to pan with tomato purée and water.
- Cover and cook for a further 5–10 minutes.
- Serve with rice and green vegetables.

Nutritional information (per serving):
Calories = 657; protein = 58 g; carbohydrate = 74 g; fat = 16.1 g; fibre = 2.2 g

Rice, Bean and Vegetable Stir Fry

Serves 2

6 oz (175 g) brown rice
1 tbsp olive oil
1 onion, chopped
2 cloves garlic, crushed
1 piece fresh root ginger, chopped

4 oz (100 g) large mushrooms, sliced
2 stalks celery, chopped
4 oz (100 g) peas
Half a 15 oz (400 g) can red kidney beans

- ◆ Cover rice with plenty of boiling water.
- ◆ Bring to the boil and simmer for 25–30 minutes.
- ◆ Meanwhile, heat oil in a wok over a high heat.
- ◆ Add the onion, and stir fry for 1 minute.
- ◆ Add garlic, ginger, mushrooms, celery and peas, and stir fry for 3 minutes.
- ◆ Tip in red kidney beans and cooked rice.
- ◆ Cook for a further 2 minutes, until all ingredients are thoroughly heated through.

Nutritional information (per serving):
Calories = 526; protein = 18.3 g; carbohydrate = 94.2 g; fat = 11.3 g; fibre = 11.1 g

Vegetarian Chilli Con Carne

Serves 2

1 clove garlic, crushed
1 onion, chopped
1 green or red pepper, chopped
½ tsp chilli powder (or to taste)
8 oz (225 g) can tomatoes

2 oz (50 g) red lentils
½ pint (300 ml) water
6 oz (175 g) rice
½ of a 14 oz (400 g) can red kidney beans

- ◆ Place garlic, onion, pepper, chilli, tomatoes, lentils, water and rice in a large pan.
- ◆ Bring to the boil and simmer for 20 minutes.
- ◆ Add drained kidney beans and cook for a further 5 minutes.
- ◆ Season to taste.
- ◆ Serve with broccoli or green salad.

Nutritional information (per serving):
Calories = 550; protein = 21 g; carbohydrate = 119 g; fat = 2.3 g; fibre = 10.4 g

Rice Salad

This salad can be served as a main course. The vegetables can be varied according to what is at hand.

Serves 2

6 oz (175 g) rice
2 spring onions, chopped
½ red pepper and ½ green
  pepper, chopped
4 oz (100 g) can tuna (in brine or
  water), drained, *or*
2 hard boiled eggs, chopped, *or*

½ of a 14 oz (400 g) can red
  kidney beans *or*
4 oz (100 g) cooked chicken or
  turkey, chopped, *or*
2 oz (50 g) peanuts
2 oz (50 g) raisins or chopped
  dates

For the dressing:

2 tbsp (30 ml) olive oil
1 tsp (5 ml) wine vinegar

1 tsp (5 ml) orange juice

◆ Cook rice, and mix with vegetables, raisins or dates and tuna.
◆ Shake ingredients for dressing together.
◆ Combine with salad.

Nutritional information (per serving):
Calories = 598; protein = 20 g; carbohydrate = 97 g; fat = 16.7 g; fibre = 2.2 g

V Bulgar Wheat and Lentil Pilaff

Bulgar wheat has a slightly nutty flavour and can be used instead of rice for most dishes. It is very easy to cook, and is available from most health food shops and supermarkets.

Serves 2

6 oz (175 g) bulgar wheat
¾ pint (450 ml) boiling water
1 small onion, chopped
1 small green pepper, chopped
2 carrots, sliced

1 tbsp (15 ml) concentrated
  vegetable stock (e.g. Vecon) *or*
1 vegetable stock cube
4 oz (100 g) green lentils, pre-
  soaked in water

◆ Cover the bulgar wheat with the boiling water and leave to stand for 20 minutes.
◆ Meanwhile, place the remaining ingredients in a large pan.
◆ Bring to the boil, cover and simmer for 30 minutes, until the lentils are soft. (In a pressure cooker, reduce cooking time to 7 minutes, and release steam slowly.)
◆ Spoon bulgar wheat onto a serving plate and top with lentil mixture.

Nutritional information (per serving):
Calories = 489; protein = 22 g; carbohydrate = 98 g; fat = 2.8 g; fibre = 6.2 g

Pilaff with Plaice

Serves 2

6 oz (175 g) brown rice
1 pint (600 ml) water
1 small onion, chopped
Pinch of turmeric (or mild curry
    powder)
1 courgette
1 small red pepper

12 oz (350 g) plaice fillets, cut into
    strips
Salt and freshly ground black
    pepper
1 tbsp (15 ml) sunflower seeds
    (optional)

♦ Place rice, water, onion and turmeric in a large saucepan.
♦ Bring to the boil, cover and simmer for 20 minutes.
♦ Add courgette, red pepper, plaice and seasoning.
♦ Cook for a further 5 minutes or until fish is cooked and water absorbed.
♦ Scatter sunflower seeds over before serving.

Nutritional information (per serving):
Calories = 530; protein = 40 g; carbohydrate = 76 g; fat = 9.5 g; fibre = 3.1 g

Couscous with Fish Stew

Couscous is available from health food shops partly cooked, and requires very little further cooking. It fluffs up to produce a huge amount – a little certainly goes a long way. It is excellent with a little dried fruit, such as raisins or dates, and can also be used to accompany a hearty stew.

Serves 2

6 oz (175 g) couscous
½ of a 14 oz (400 g) tin chick peas
1 oz (25 g) raisins
12 oz (350 g) white fish (e.g.
    haddock, sea bass or cod)

1 large onion, roughly chopped
¾ pint (450 ml) water
8 oz (225 g) vegetables (e.g.
    carrots or celery)
1 tsp (5 ml) mixed herbs

♦ Place couscous in a bowl and cover with boiling water.
♦ Leave to stand for 20 minutes, to absorb water.
♦ Then, mix in chick peas and raisins.
♦ Meanwhile, place all ingredients for fish stew in a large saucepan.
♦ Bring to the boil, cover and simmer for 15 minutes.
♦ Place couscous on a plate and top with fish stew.

Nutritional information (per serving):
Calories = 548; protein = 49 g; carbohydrate = 78 g; fat = 6 g; fibre = 7.1 g

Couscous aux Sept Legumes

For an authentic Moroccan dish, make a vegetable stew with couscous, as follows.

Serves 2

1 lb (450 g) mixed vegetables (choose 7 varieties, e.g. carrots, aubergines, potatoes, broad beans, French beans, courgettes, mushrooms)

¼ pint (150 ml) water
1 tbsp (15 ml) concentrated vegetable stock (e.g. Vecon) *or* 1 vegetable stock cube

♦ Leave couscous to stand in a bowl of boiling water, in which the stock is dissolved, for 20 minutes.
♦ Then bring vegetables to the boil, cover and simmer for 15 minutes.
♦ Serve with couscous.

Nutritional information (per serving):
Calories = 435; protein = 14.9 g; carbohydrate = 89 g; fat = 4.6 g; fibre = 9.3 g

Pasta and noodles

Pasta is made from durum wheat flour and water or egg. It is an excellent source of carbohydrate and has a lower glycaemic index than other cereals. Pasta is also very quick to cook: usually 10 minutes for dried types and 2–4 minutes for fresh. It can form the basis of many healthy, low fat meals. Wholemeal varieties are higher in fibre and are therefore more filling. Top pasta shapes with one of the following sauces for a quick, nourishing meal.

Lentil Sauce

Serves 2

1 onion, chopped
1 clove garlic, crushed
8 oz (225 g) tin tomatoes

4 oz (100 g) red lentils
1 pint (600 ml) water
1 tsp (5 ml) oregano

♦ Place all ingredients in a large pan.
♦ Bring to the boil, cover and simmer for 20 minutes. (Alternatively, cook in a pressure cooker for 3 minutes.)

Nutritional information (per serving):
Calories = 177; protein = 13 g; carbohydrate = 31.5 g; fat = 0.8 g; fibre = 3.2 g

V

Easy Tomato Sauce

Serves 2

1 onion, chopped
1 clove garlic, crushed
14 oz (400 g) tin tomatoes
1 tsp (5 ml) oregano
1 tbsp (15 ml) tomato purée

Dash of tabasco
2 tsp (10 ml) parmesan cheese
Freshly ground black pepper and
    salt, to taste

◆ Place all ingredients in a large pan, bring to the boil and simmer for 5–10 minutes. (Liquidise for a smoother sauce.)
◆ Top with parmesan cheese, and serve with salad.

Nutritional information (per serving):
Calories = 37; protein = 2.3 g; carbohydrate = 7 g; fat = 0.2 g; fibre = 1.6 g

Salmon and Broccoli Sauce

Serves 2

6 oz (175 g) broccoli florets
½ pint (300 ml) skimmed *or*
    semi-skimmed milk
1 tbsp (15 ml) cornflour

7 oz (200 g) tin salmon, drained
    and flaked
2 tsp (10 ml) parmesan cheese
Freshly ground black pepper

◆ Cook broccoli in a small amount of boiling water for 7 minutes, and drain.
◆ Mix together milk and cornflour.
◆ Heat gently until thickened (can be done in a microwave oven).
◆ Stir in broccoli and salmon.
◆ Serve topped with parmesan cheese and black pepper.

Nutritional information (per serving):
Calories = 283; protein = 31.1 g; carbohydrate = 16 g; fat = 10.8 g; fibre = 2.3 g

'Creamy' Chicken Sauce

Serves 2

8 oz (225 g) cooked chicken,
    chopped
8 oz (225 g) fromage frais (8% fat)

1 tbsp (15 ml) lemon juice
Freshly ground black pepper
Fresh parsley, chopped

◆ Combine chicken, fromage frais, lemon juice and black pepper.
◆ Heat gently, not quite to boiling point (otherwise the sauce will curdle). Sprinkle with parsley, and serve with green salad.

Nutritional information (per serving):
Calories = 311; protein = 41.1 g; carbohydrate = 6.4 g; fat = 13.5 g; fibre = 0 g

V

Tomato and Aubergine Sauce

Serves 2

2 tsp (10 ml) olive oil
1 quantity easy tomato sauce (see page 198)

1 small aubergine, cubed
2 tsp (10 ml) parmesan *or* cottage cheese

- Cook the aubergine in the oil for 10 minutes.
- Stir in the tomato sauce, and serve with a little parmesan or cottage cheese.

Nutritional information (per serving):
Calories = 102; protein = 3.5 g; carbohydrate = 9.8 g; fat = 5.7 g; fibre = 4.2 g

Noodles with Prawns and Green Beans

Serves 2

8 oz (225 g) frozen whole green beans
6 oz (175 g) egg noodles

1 tsp (5 ml) oil
6 oz (175 g) peeled prawns
1 tbsp (15 ml) soy sauce

- Cook green beans in a little boiling water for 5 minutes, then drain.
- Cook noodles in a large pan for 10 minutes.
- Meanwhile, heat oil in a wok or frying pan and stir fry prawns for 2 minutes.
- Add beans, noodles and soy sauce, and heat through.

Nutritional information (per serving):
Calories = 483; protein = 32.4 g; carbohydrate = 66 g; fat = 11.8 g; fibre = 5.2 g

V

Mushroom Pasta

Serves 2

4 oz (100 g) mushrooms
2 tsp (10 ml) olive oil
1 onion, sliced

½ green pepper, sliced
2 tbsp (30 ml) fromage frais (8% fat)
6 oz (175 g) pasta shapes

- Either leave mushrooms whole or, if quite large, roughly slice.
- Heat oil in a pan and cook onion and pepper for 5 minutes.
- Add mushrooms and continue cooking for 5 minutes.
- Remove from heat and stir in fromage frais. Do not boil.
- Meanwhile, cook pasta for about 10 minutes in boiling water.
- Drain and combine with the mushroom sauce.
- Serve with green salad.

Nutritional information (per serving):
Calories = 438; protein = 13.6 g; carbohydrate = 71 g; fat = 13 g; fibre = 3.7 g

Seafood Tagliatelle

Serves 2

1 tsp (5 ml) oil
1 small onion, sliced
½ oz (15 g) flour
¼ pint (150 ml) low fat milk
3 tbsp (45 ml) water *or* white wine

Freshly ground black pepper
2 oz (50 g) mushrooms, sliced
8 oz (225 g) haddock fillet, cubed
2 oz (50 g) peeled prawns
6 oz (175 g) tagliatelle

- Heat oil in a pan and cook onion until soft.
- Stir in flour and cook for 1 minute.
- Remove from heat and gradually stir in milk.
- Return to heat and cook, stirring all the time, until thickened and smooth.
- Add water or white wine, black pepper, mushrooms and haddock fillet.
- Simmer for about 5 minutes.
- Stir in prawns and cook for a further 1–2 minutes until the prawns are hot.
- Meanwhile, cook and drain tagliatelle, then combine with seafood sauce.

Nutritional information (per serving):
Calories = 507; protein = 45.2 g; carbohydrate = 73 g; fat = 5.7 g; fibre = 3.2 g

V

Tofu with Noodles

Serves 2

For the marinade:

2 tbsp (30 ml) soy sauce
2 tbsp (30 ml) dry sherry

1 tbsp (15 ml) wine vinegar

For the dish:

8 oz (225 g) tofu (bean curd), cubed
1 tbsp (15 ml) olive oil
1 clove garlic, crushed
1 piece fresh root ginger, chopped

1 red pepper, sliced
4 oz (100 g) mange tout
1 tsp (5 ml) cornflour
6 oz (175 g) noodles, cooked in water

- Mix ingredients for marinade together.
- Add tofu and leave for at least 30 minutes in fridge (or overnight).
- Heat oil in a wok and stir fry the garlic, ginger and vegetables for 4 minutes.
- Remove tofu from marinade.

◆ Blend marinade with cornflour, and pour over the vegetables.
◆ Stir until sauce has thickened.
◆ Place vegetables and sauce in a serving dish.
◆ Stir fry tofu for 2 minutes, and add to vegetables.
◆ Serve with noodles.

Nutritional information (per serving):
Calories = 533; protein = 21 g; carbohydrate = 75 g; fat = 18.5 g; fibre = 3.8 g

Potatoes

Potatoes are excellent sources of complex carbohydrate. They also provide vitamin C and fibre, and are a good basis for all meals.

Baked potatoes

Baked potatoes are quick to cook if you have a microwave – about 10 minutes is enough for one large potato. If you are cooking with a conventional oven, save time by cooking several potatoes at once. Wrap in foil, and bake for about one hour. Allow them to cool and keep them in the fridge. They will last for up to a week.

Here are some recipes for quick and nutritious toppings. Simply cut the potato in half and spoon the topping over. Serve with a salad or vegetables.

Mexican Tuna Filling

Serves 1

4 oz (100 g) tin tuna, drained
2 tbsp (30 ml) tinned red kidney
  beans

2 tbsp (30 ml) sweetcorn
Dash of tabasco (chilli) sauce

◆ Combine all ingredients in a saucepan.
◆ Heat through.

Nutritional information (per serving):
Calories = 247; protein = 34 g; carbohydrate = 22 g; fat = 2.8 g; fibre = 5 g

Chick Pea Filling

Serves 1

Half an onion
½ tsp (2.5 ml) coriander and
  cumin, *or* curry powder

¼ of a 14 oz (400 g) can chick
  peas, drained
2 tbsp (30 ml) plain yoghurt

- Scoop out flesh from potato, keeping skin intact.
- Blend flesh and ingredients in food processor until almost smooth, or mash with a fork.
- Pile filling back in potato skin.
- Heat through again.

Nutritional information (per serving):
Calories = 149; protein = 10.3 g; carbohydrate = 21 g; fat = 3.4 g; fibre = 4.1 g

Peanut and Yoghurt Filling

Serves 1

1 tbsp (15 ml) crunchy peanut
  butter

2 tbsp (30 ml) plain yoghurt

- Scoop out some of potato flesh and mash with peanut butter and yoghurt.
- Pile back into skin.
- Heat through.

Nutritional information (per serving):
Calories = 183; protein = 8.5 g; carbohydrate = 7.6 g; fat = 13.4 g; fibre = 1.3 g

Chicken and Sweetcorn Filling

Serves 1

4 oz (100 g) cooked chicken,
  chopped

3 tbsp (45 ml) sweetcorn
2 tbsp (30 ml) cottage cheese

- Combine chicken, sweetcorn and cottage cheese.
- Serve hot or cold.

Nutritional information (per serving):
Calories = 322; protein = 42 g; carbohydrate = 18.9 g; fat = 9.3 g; fibre = 2 g

Potato and Fish Pie

Serves 2

1 lb (450 g) potatoes
7 oz (200 g) white fish fillets
  (e.g. cod or plaice)
3 tbsp (45 ml) skimmed milk

2 eggs
1 tbsp (15 ml) parsley
1 tbsp (15 ml) lemon juice

- Cut potatoes into chunks and boil until tender.
- Drain, then mash with flaked fish, milk, eggs, parsley and lemon juice.
- Place in a dish, then cook either in microwave at full power for 5 minutes, or in oven at 200°C/400°F/gas mark 6 for 20 minutes.
- Serve with green vegetables.

Nutritional information (per serving):
Calories = 352; protein = 33.3 g; carbohydrate = 39.4 g; fat = 7.9 g; fibre = 2.8 g

V

Cheese and Potato Layer

Serves 2

1 lb (450 g) potatoes, thinly sliced
1 large onion, cut into thin rings
4 oz (100 g) half fat Cheddar
  cheese, grated

1 tsp (5 ml) herbs (e.g. sage or
  thyme)
¼ pint (150 ml) skimmed milk
Freshly ground black pepper

- In a dish, layer potatoes, onion, cheese, black pepper and herbs, finishing with a layer of cheese.
- Pour milk over the dish and cover.
- Cook either in microwave at full power for 15 minutes or in oven at 200°C/400°F/gas mark 6 for 1 hour.
- Serve with vegetables or salad.

Nutritional information (per serving):
Calories = 479; protein = 27.6 g; carbohydrate = 79 g; fat = 8.1 g; fibre = 6.8 g

V

Spicy Potatoes with Courgettes

Serves 2

1 lb (450 g) small new potatoes
4 oz (100 g) cauliflower, broken
  into florets
1 tbsp (15 ml) oil

1 onion, sliced
2 tsp (10 ml) mild curry powder
Pinch chilli powder
3 courgettes, sliced

- Boil potatoes in their skins and cauliflower for 10 minutes, then drain.
- Meanwhile, heat oil in a wok or heavy based pan, and stir fry onion and spices for 3 minutes.

- Add courgettes and stir fry for a further 2 minutes.
- Add potatoes and cauliflower and cook for a further 3 minutes or until heated through.

Follow this dish with a high protein dessert, such as yoghurt or cheesecake (*see* pages 209–213).

Nutritional information (per serving):
Calories = 278; protein = 7.1 g; carbohydrate = 45 g; fat = 9 g; fibre = 4.5 g

V   Spanish Potato Omelette

Serves 2

1 lb (450 g) potatoes   6 eggs
1 tsp (5 ml) oil   Salt and black pepper
1 onion, chopped   Paprika

- Boil potatoes in their skins.
- Cool and cut into thick slices.
- Cook onion in oil for 5 minutes, then add potatoes.
- Beat eggs with salt and pepper and pour into the pan with vegetables.
- Sprinkle with paprika. Lower heat and cook for about 5 minutes until nearly set.
- Finish off under a hot grill for 1–2 minutes or until top sets.
- Serve with tomato salad.

Nutritional information (per serving):
Calories = 458; protein = 27 g; carbohydrate = 40 g; fat = 22 g; fibre = 3.1 g

Beans and lentils

Beans and lentils supply protein, fibre and a wide range of important vitamins and minerals. You can buy them ready-cooked in tins – simply drain them, and use them in these recipes. Dried beans need soaking for several hours, although you can reduce the soaking time to just one hour if you use boiling water. Using a pressure cooker is quicker – follow the recommended times. Alternatively, boil them in a saucepan (times are given in the recipes). It is worth making a larger quantity than you need and freezing or keeping some in the fridge for a few days to save time.

Beans and lentils can be rather bland on their own, but they readily absorb the flavour of other ingredients. These recipes should give you lots of ideas for using them in exciting ways.

V

Soya Bean Curry

Soya beans are best cooked in a pressure cooker, since they require a long cooking time. The addition of sultanas gives a subtle, sweet flavour that complements the beans well.

Serves 2

6 oz (175 g) soya beans, soaked
   for several hours
1 tbsp (15 ml) curry powder
1 onion, chopped
1 clove garlic, crushed

2 carrots, sliced
2 courgettes, sliced
2 tbsp (30 ml) sultanas
1 tbsp (15 ml) tomato purée

- Drain beans and place in pressure cooker with about ½ pint (300 ml) water.
- Add curry powder and bring to the boil.
- Cook for 15 minutes.
- Release steam slowly, then add remaining ingredients.
- Bring to the boil and cook for a further 3 minutes, before releasing steam slowly.
- Serve with baked potatoes.

Nutritional information (per serving):
Calories = 396; protein = 33 g; carbohydrate = 31 g; fat = 16.6 g; fibre = 16.2 g

Chicken with Chick Peas and Apricots

Chicken with apricots sounds an unusual combination, but it tastes delicious and supplies lots of valuable nutrients. Apricots are high in beta carotene (vitamin A).

Serves 2

1 tsp (5 ml) oil
1 onion, chopped
1 piece fresh root ginger, finely
   chopped
2 chicken breasts, cut into large
   pieces

2 cloves garlic, crushed
3 oz (75 g) dried, ready-to-eat
   apricots
¼ pint (150 ml) water
14 oz (400 g) tin chick peas

- Heat oil in a wok or a heavy based pan.
- Stir fry onion, garlic, ginger and chicken for about 4 minutes.
- Add apricots, water and chick peas.
- Simmer for 15 minutes.
- Serve with boiled rice and green vegetables.

Nutritional information (per serving):
Calories = 502; protein = 47 g; carbohydrate = 52 g; fat = 13.3 g; fibre = 11.6 g

V

Mixed Bean Hotpot

Serves 2

14 oz (400 g) can of beans (e.g. red kidney beans, chick peas or haricot beans)
4 oz (100 g) green beans
8 oz (225 g) can tomatoes

1 tbsp (15 ml) tomato purée
1 tsp (5 ml) mixed herbs
1 lb (450 g) potatoes, boiled and cooled

- Place drained can of beans in large casserole dish and mix in green beans, tomatoes, purée and herbs.
- Thinly slice potatoes and arrange on top.
- Bake at 170°C/325°F/gas mark 3 for 30 minutes until the potatoes are cooked, or microwave on full for 8 minutes, turning frequently.
- Serve with green vegetables or salad.

Nutritional information (per serving):
Calories = 346; protein = 16.8 g; carbohydrate = 71 g; fat = 1.5 g; fibre = 14.2 g

V

Pasta and Chick Pea Salad

The combination of chick peas and pasta is wonderful. This dish is simple to make, using mostly store cupboard ingredients. Vary the vegetables according to what is at hand.

Serves 2

6 oz (175 g) pasta twists
4 oz (100 g) peas
4 oz (100 g) sweetcorn
4 oz (100 g) canned pineapple

½ red pepper, diced
8 oz (225 g) cooked chick peas
4 oz (100 g) fromage frais

- Cook pasta for 10 minutes.
- Drain and combine with remaining ingredients.

Nutritional information (per serving):
Calories = 576; protein = 28 g; carbohydrate = 109 g; fat = 6.5 g; fibre = 11.6 g

V

Lentil and Vegetable Lasagne

This lasagne has a fluffy, light topping and is lower in fat than the traditional version. It is a very impressive dish when entertaining. If you are in a hurry, simply top with fromage frais.

Serves 2

6 sheets ready-cooked lasagne

For the lentil and vegetable sauce:

4 oz (100 g) red lentils
1 onion, chopped
14 oz (400 g) tin of tomatoes

2 carrots, chopped
1 tsp (5 ml) oregano
¼ pint (150 ml) water

For the topping:

4 oz (100 g) fromage frais
2 eggs

1 tbsp (15 ml) parmesan cheese

◆ Place all ingredients for lentil and vegetable sauce in a saucepan and bring to the boil.
◆ Simmer for 20 minutes or cook in pressure cooker for 3 minutes (release steam slowly).
◆ Place half of the sauce in a dish, with several lasagne sheets on top. Then add rest of sauce, followed by remaining lasagne sheets. For topping, beat eggs with fromage frais, then spoon them on top of lasagne. Sprinkle with parmesan cheese. Bake at 200°C/400°F/gas mark 6 for 40 minutes, until the topping is golden. Serve with large mixed salad.

Nutritional information (per serving):
Calories = 513; protein = 33 g; carbohydrate = 75 g; fat = 10.9 g; fibre = 6 g

V   **Lentil and Vegetable Stew**

Cooking this dish in a pressure cooker saves a lot of time. You can substitute red lentils or beans for green lentils.

Serves 2

4 oz (100 g) green lentils, soaked
   for a few hours
1 tbsp (15 ml) concentrated
   vegetable stock (e.g. Vecon), *or*
1 vegetable stock cube
½ pint (300 ml) water

1 onion, chopped
2 carrots
1 red or green pepper, sliced
1 potato, chopped
2 courgettes

◆ Drain lentils and place in pressure cooker (or a large saucepan) with vegetable stock and water.
◆ Bring to the boil and cook for 10 minutes.
◆ Release steam, then add vegetables.
◆ Bring back to the boil and cook for a further 3 minutes, then release steam slowly.
◆ Serve with boiled or baked potatoes.

Nutritional information (per serving):
Calories = 232; protein = 15.2 g; carbohydrate = 42 g; fat = 1.7 g; fibre = 8.2 g

V

Lentil Loaf

This loaf is surprisingly easy to make and looks impressive. It is also extremely low in fat. Cut any leftovers into slices and use as a sandwich filling.

Serves 4

4 oz (100 g) red lentils
1 onion, chopped
1 tbsp (15 ml) concentrated
   vegetable stock (e.g. Vecon), *or*
1 vegetable stock cube

½ pint (300 ml) water
2 oz (50 g) oats or fresh
   breadcrumbs
1 egg, beaten

◆ Place lentils, onion, stock concentrate and water in a large pan.
◆ Bring to the boil and simmer for 20 minutes, or cook in pressure cooker for 3 minutes and release steam slowly.
◆ Stir in oats or breadcrumbs, and egg.
◆ Spoon into 1 lb (450 g) non-stick loaf tin.
◆ Cover with foil and bake at 190°C/375°F/gas mark 5 for 30 minutes.
◆ Leave in the tin for 2 minutes, then loosen and turn out.
◆ Serve with rice and vegetables.

Nutritional information (per serving):
Calories = 321; protein = 19.4 g; carbohydrate = 50 g; fat = 6.1 g; fibre = 4.9 g

V

Bean Burgers

These are much lower in fat than beef burgers. Make a large batch, so that you can keep some in the freezer for when you are in a hurry.

Serves 2

14 oz (400 g) tin red kidney beans,
   drained
2 tsp (10 ml) oil
1 small onion, finely chopped

1 clove garlic, crushed
1 tbsp (15 ml) parsley
1 tbsp (15 ml) lemon juice
Oats for coating

◆ Cook the onion and garlic in the oil for 5 minutes.
◆ Mash with a fork or blend in food processor with other ingredients, except the oats, till a coarse purée.
◆ Add a little flour if necessary for a firmer texture.
◆ Place oats in a dish.
◆ In your hands, form mixture into 4 large burgers, coating them with oats.
◆ Grill for about 2 minutes on each side, fry in a small amount of hot oil, or barbecue.
◆ Serve in a wholemeal bap or pitta bread with lots of salad.

Nutritional information (2 burgers):
Calories = 234; protein = 11.6 g; carbohydrate = 34 g; fat = 6.6 g; fibre = 10.2 g

Puddings and desserts

Puddings and desserts can make a substantial nutritional contribution to diet. They need not be full of sugar or dripping in cream. They can, in fact, be very healthy if based on fruit and low fat ingredients like yoghurt and fromage frais.

These desserts and puddings are all easy to make. If you really are pressed for time, fresh fruit and yoghurt are always a good choice. If you have a little longer or are entertaining, these recipes will help to add a new dimension to your diet!

Apricot and Lemon Mousse

You can use other dried fruits such as peaches or prunes in this recipe instead of apricots, if you wish.

Serves 2

4 oz (100 g) dried apricots   Juice and rind of 1 lemon
½ pint (300 ml) orange juice   8 oz (225 g) plain fromage frais

- Soak apricots in orange juice in a bowl overnight.
- In a liquidiser or food processor, blend them into a purée.
- Add remaining ingredients and blend until smooth.
- Spoon into glasses.
- Chill in the fridge before serving.

Nutritional information (per serving):
Calories = 221; protein = 12.9 g; carbohydrate = 44.3 g; fat = 0.3 g; fibre = 3.8 g

Banana and Oat Pudding

Serves 2

2 ripe bananas   ½ pint (300 ml) plain yoghurt
1 oz (25 g) porridge oats

- Mash one banana with oats and yoghurt.
- Put the mixture into individual bowls.
- Decorate with remaining banana, cut into slices.

Nutritional information (per serving):
Calories = 213; protein = 10.3 g; carbohydrate = 40 g; fat = 2.6 g; fibre = 2 g

Banana Pancakes

Makes 8 pancakes

4 oz (100 g) wholemeal flour, or
fine oatmeal
½ pint (300 ml) skimmed or semi-
skimmed milk

2 eggs
1 tsp (5 ml) oil
3 ripe bananas

◆ Blend all ingredients, except bananas, in a liquidiser for 30 seconds.
◆ Then heat a non-stick frying pan and add oil.
◆ Pour in 1 tablespoonful of batter, tilting the pan to coat evenly.
◆ Cook until underside of pancake is brown.
◆ Turn, and cook for a further 10 seconds until other side is brown.
◆ Repeat till batter used up.
◆ Stack pancakes on an oven proof plate and keep warm in the oven on a very low heat.
◆ Then, mix one mashed banana with two sliced bananas.
◆ Place spoonful on each pancake and fold into quarters.
◆ Serve with low fat yoghurt.

Nutritional information (per pancake):
Calories = 103; protein = 5.1 g; carbohydrate = 17.1 g; fat = 2 g; fibre = 1.5 g

Baked Apples

Make this pudding in the autumn, when apples are cheap.

Serves 1

1 large cooking apple
1 tbsp (15 ml) raisins *or* sultanas
1 tsp (5 ml) honey

1 tsp (5 ml) toasted, chopped
hazelnuts (optional)

◆ Remove core from apple.
◆ Score skin lightly around middle. Place in small dish. Mix together raisins or sultanas, honey and nuts and fill centre of apple.
◆ Cover loosely with foil and bake at 180°C/350°F/gas mark 4 for 45–60 minutes *or* cover with another dish and microwave on medium power for 5–7 minutes (depending on the size of apple).
◆ Serve with yoghurt, low fat custard or fromage frais.

Nutritional information (per serving):
Calories = 144; protein = 1.2 g; carbohydrate = 33 g; fat = 1.8 g; fibre = 0.6 g

Chocolate and Banana Cheesecake

Makes 8 slices

For the base:

1 oz (25 g) margarine *or* butter
2 tbsp (30 ml) honey

2 oz (50 g) milk chocolate
4 oz (100 g) oatmeal

For the cheesecake:

2 ripe bananas, chopped
8 oz (225 g) fromage frais
2 tbsp (30 ml) honey

4 tbsp (60 ml) plain yoghurt
2 eggs

◆ For base, melt margarine, honey and chocolate in small bowl in microwave or saucepan.
◆ Do not allow to boil.
◆ Stir in the oatmeal.
◆ Press into base of 8″ microwave cake dish or loose-bottomed cake tin.
◆ Blend cheesecake ingredients in liquidiser for 1 minute.
◆ Pour onto the base.
◆ Cook, either in the microwave on medium power for 20 minutes, or in conventional oven at 325°F/160°C/gas mark 3 for 1–1½ hours.
◆ Cool and decorate with grated chocolate, if you wish.

Nutritional information (per slice):
Calories = 194; protein = 7.2 g; carbohydrate = 26 g; fat = 7.4 g; fibre = 1.1 g

Tropical Fruit Salad

Exotic fruits are available all year round now in supermarkets. They are packed with vitamins A and C.

Serves 2

1 mango (or paw paw)
1 orange
1 banana

1 kiwi fruit
4 rings fresh or tinned pineapple
¼ pint (150 ml) orange juice

◆ Peel and chop mango, orange, banana and kiwi fruit.
◆ Mix with pineapple and orange juice.
◆ Keep in fridge before serving to preserve vitamins.

Nutritional information (per serving):
Calories = 220; protein = 2.7 g; carbohydrate = 56 g; fat = 0.2 g; fibre = 7 g

Wholemeal Bread and Butter Pudding

This pudding is great for athletes, as it is high in complex carbohydrates from the bread, and has lots of protein, calcium and B vitamins from the milk. It is worth making a larger quantity that you need, as it will keep in the fridge for several days.

Serves 4

8 slices wholemeal bread
1½ oz (40 g) low fat spread
3 oz (75 g) sultanas
1 tbsp (15 ml) brown sugar

3 eggs
1 pint (600 ml) skimmed milk
Nutmeg

- Spread bread with low fat spread.
- Cut each slice into 4 squares and put in 2 pint (1 l) dish.
- Scatter sultanas between each slice.
- Beat together sugar, eggs, and milk and pour over bread.
- Sprinkle with a little grated nutmeg.
- Leave to soak for 30 minutes, if time allows.
- Bake at 350°F/180°C/gas mark 4 for 1 hour, until the top is golden.

Nutritional information (per serving):
Calories = 345; protein = 17 g; carbohydrate = 49 g; fat = 10.5 g; fibre = 3.9 g

Raisin and Lemon Ice Cream

This ice cream is easy to make, low in fat and quite delicious!

Makes 4 servings

2 oz (50 g) raisins
Juice of 1 lemon

8 fl oz (250 ml) evaporated milk
2 oz (50 g) castor sugar

- Soak raisins in lemon juice for 2 hours.
- Whisk evaporated milk until foamy and holding its shape.
- Whisk in sugar.
- Stir in raisins and lemon juice.
- Freeze in ice cream maker or shallow container, whisking once or twice.

Nutritional information (per serving):
Calories = 178; protein = 5.5 g; carbohydrate = 27 g; fat = 5.9 g; fibre = 0.3 g

Banana Yoghurt Ice Cream

Makes 4 servings

2 ripe bananas
2 tbsp (30 ml) honey

8 fl oz (250 ml) plain yoghurt
1 tbsp lemon juice

◆ Blend ingredients in liquidiser until smooth.
◆ Freeze in ice cream maker or shallow container, whisking once or twice.

Nutritional information (per serving):
Calories = 139; protein = 7.0 g; carbohydrate = 27 g; fat = 1.2 g; fibre = 0.6 g

Snacks – muffins, breads and cookies

These recipes for homemade, high energy snacks are not only low in fat and highly nutritious, but they are simple and quick to make (even if you have never baked before!). Make a large batch, wrap in foil and take in your kit bag so you'll never be stuck for snacks before or after training again.

Oatbran and Raisin Muffins

High in carbohydrate and soluble fibre but very low in fat, these muffins are delicious and simple to make. Try some of the numerous variations below!

Makes 12 muffins

8 oz (225 g) oatbran
1 tbsp (15 ml) baking powder
1 tsp (5 ml) cinnamon
2 oz (50 g) brown sugar or honey

1 tbsp (15 ml) oil
2 egg whites
2 oz (50 g) raisins
12 fl oz (350 ml) skimmed milk

◆ Combine oatbran, baking powder and sugar.
◆ Stir in remaining ingredients.
◆ Leave to stand for a few minutes to allow some of liquid to absorb.
◆ Spoon into 12 non stick bun tins (or paper cases).
◆ Bake at 220°C/425°F/gas mark 7 for 12–15 minutes.

Nutritional information (per muffin):
Calories = 123; protein = 4.6 g; carbohydrate = 20 g; fat = 2.8 g; fibre = 3.6 g

Variations:

- Substitute 1 grated apple for the raisins.
- Add 2 oz (50 g) dates and 2 oz (50 g) walnuts instead of the raisins. Omit the cinnamon.
- Substitute 4 oz (100 g) tinned black cherries (pitted) for the raisins. Omit the cinnamon.
- Substitute 8 oz (225 g) tinned crushed pineapple in juice (drained) for the raisins. Omit the cinnamon.
- Substitute 2 mashed bananas for the raisins. Omit the cinnamon.

Banana Muffins

These heavenly muffins can be varied according to the fruit available.

Makes 10 muffins

2 oz (50 g) butter
3 oz (75 g) brown sugar
1 egg
8 oz (225 g) flour (wholemeal or
  half wholemeal, half white)

2 mashed bananas
Pinch salt
1 tsp (5 ml) baking powder
1 tsp (5 ml) vanilla essence
5 tbsp (75 ml) skimmed milk

- Combine all ingredients in a large bowl.
- Spoon into 10 non stick bun tins (or paper cases).
- Bake at 190°C/375°F/gas mark 5 for approx 20 minutes.

Nutritional information (per muffin):
Calories = 164; protein = 4.1 g; carbohydrate = 27 g; fat = 5.3 g; fibre = 2.2 g

Variations:

- Add 2 oz (50 g) chocolate chips to the mixture (recommended!).
- Substitute 8 oz (225 g) fresh blueberries or 3 oz (75 g) dried blueberries for the bananas.
- Substitute 8 oz (225 g) fresh cranberries or 3 oz (75 g) dried cranberries for the bananas. Add 2 oz (50 g) chopped walnuts.
- Substitute 4 oz (100 g) chopped dried apricots for the bananas. Add the grated rind of 1 lemon instead of the vanilla essence.

Peanut Butter Muffins

Peanut butter is simply ground peanuts with a little salt and is therefore an excellent source of unsaturated fatty acids, zinc, protein and fibre. If you have a weakness for peanut butter, these muffins won't last long!

Makes 10 muffins

4 oz (100 g) crunchy peanut butter
4 oz (100 g) honey
2 eggs
1 tsp (5 ml) vanilla essence

8 oz (225 g) half wholemeal, half
  white self raising flour
3–4 tbsp (45–60 ml) milk
1 oz (25 g) plain peanuts

- ◆ Combine peanut butter and honey.
- ◆ Add eggs, vanilla essence, flour and milk.
- ◆ Spoon into 10 non stick bun tins.
- ◆ Press a few peanuts on top of each muffin.
- ◆ Bake at 190°C/375°F/gas mark 5 for 25 minutes.

Nutritional information (per muffin):
Calories = 192; protein = 7.1 g; carbohydrate = 24 g; fat = 8.2 g; fibre = 2.2 g

Cornmeal Muffins

Yellow cornmeal (polenta) gives a moreish, soft texture to these unusual muffins. A little lower in fibre than wholemeal flour but higher than white flour, cornmeal is good for iron, B vitamins and carbohydrate.

Makes 12 muffins

6 oz (175 g) cornmeal
2 oz (50 g) self raising white
  flour
1 tbsp (15 ml) baking powder
2 tbsp (30 ml) honey

2 oz (50 g) sultanas
1 tsp (5 ml) vanilla essence
2 egg whites
10 fl oz (300 ml) skimmed milk
2 tbsp (30 ml) oil or melted butter

- ◆ Mix all ingredients together in a bowl. (Batter should be fairly runny as cornmeal absorbs a lot of liquid during cooking.)
- ◆ Spoon into 12 non stick bun tins (or paper cases).
- ◆ Bake at 400°C/200°F/gas mark 6 for 15 minutes.

Nutritional information (per muffin):
Calories = 126; protein = 3.2 g; carbohydrate = 22 g; fat = 3.1 g; fibre = 0.5 g

Variations:

- – Substitute 8 oz (225 g) fresh or 3 oz (75 g) dried cranberries for the sultanas.
- – Substitute 2 oz (50 g) chopped dates for the sultanas.
- – Add 1 tbsp (15 ml) carob powder or cocoa powder to the mixture.
- – Substitute 2 oz (50 g) glace cherries for the sultanas.

Oatmeal Biscuits

Makes 24

3 oz (75 g) wholemeal flour
5 oz (150 g) oatmeal
1 tsp (5 ml) vanilla essence
2 tbsp (30 ml) oil

2 oz (50 g) brown sugar
2 oz (50 g) chopped walnuts or
   raisins
1 egg

- ◆ Mix all ingredients together in a bowl.
- ◆ Place heaped tablespoonfuls on a non stick baking tray about 2" (5 cm) apart (they will spread while cooking).
- ◆ Bake at 180°C/350°F/gas mark 4 for 10 minutes.

Nutritional information (per biscuit):
Calories = 71; protein = 1.8 g; carbohydrate = 9 g; fat = 3.6 g; fibre = 0.8 g

Raisin Bread

Makes one loaf (10 slices)

8 oz (225 g) strong flour (half
   wholemeal, half white)
½ tsp (2.5 ml) salt
1½ tbsp (22.5 ml) sugar

1 sachet easy blend yeast
1 tbsp (15 ml) melted butter
6 fl oz (180 ml) warm water
4 oz (100 g) raisins

- ◆ Mix together flour, salt, sugar, yeast and butter.
- ◆ Add warm water to form a dough.
- ◆ Turn out onto floured surface and knead for 5–10 min.
- ◆ Knead in the raisins.
- ◆ Place in bowl, cover and leave in warm place or at room temperature to rise until doubled in size (approximately 1 hour).
- ◆ Knead for a few minutes then shape into a loaf.
- ◆ Place on oiled baking tray and bake at 220°C/425°F/gas mark 7 for 20 minutes or until it sounds hollow when tapped underneath.

Nutritional information (per slice):
Calories = 120; protein = 3.0 g; carbohydrate = 25 g; fat = 1.7 g; fibre = 1.6 g

Variations:

- – Add 2 tsp (10 ml) cinnamon to the flour mixture.
- – Substitute 4 oz (100 g) chopped dried apricots for the raisins.
- – Substitute 4 oz (100 g) sultanas for the raisins.
- – Add 1 tsp (5 ml) grated orange rind.
- – Add 2 oz (50 g) toasted chopped hazelnuts with the raisins.

Blueberry Bread

A cross between cake and bread, this recipe is a firm favourite with my family and friends!

Makes 1 large loaf (12 slices)

8 oz (225 g) strong white flour
4 oz (100 g) yellow cornmeal
1 sachet easy blend yeast
1 tsp (7.5 ml) salt
2 tbsp (30 ml) sugar

1 tbsp (22.5 ml) butter
4 oz (100 g) cottage cheese
5 tbsp (75 ml) water
8 oz (225 g) fresh or 3 oz (75 g)
   dried blueberries

- Mix all ingredients, except water and blueberries, in a bowl or combine in a food processor.
- Add water and mix until a dough forms.
- Turn out onto a floured surface and knead for 5–10 minutes.
- Knead in blueberries carefully.
- Cover and leave to rise until doubled in size.
- Knead briefly, then shape into oblong or round loaf.
- Place on oiled baking tray and bake at 220°C/425°F/gas mark 7 for approximately 20 minutes until it sounds hollow when tapped underneath.

Nutritional information (per slice):
Calories = 131; protein = 4.3 g; carbohydrate = 24 g; fat = 2.4 g; fibre = 1.4 g

Apple and Cinnamon Oat Bars

Makes 12 bars

2 apples, sliced and cooked, or 6
   oz (175 g) apple purée
6 oz (175 g) oats
2 tsp (10 ml) cinnamon

4 egg whites
1 tbsp (15 ml) honey
2 oz (50 g) raisins
6 tbsp (90 ml) skimmed milk

- Mix all ingredients together in a bowl.
- Transfer to non stick baking tin (approximately 9" × 6").
- Bake at 200°C/400°F/gas mark 6 for 15 minutes.
- When cool, cut into squares.

Nutritional information (per bar):
Calories = 87; protein = 3.1 g; carbohydrate = 17 g; fat = 1.3 g; fibre = 1.3 g

Peanut Bars

Makes 8 bars

4 tbsp (60 ml) crunchy peanut
butter
4 tbsp (60 ml) honey

8 oz (225 g) oats
2 oz (50 g) raisins
1 tbsp (15 ml) wholemeal flour

+ Melt peanut butter and honey in a saucepan.
+ Add remaining ingredients.
+ Press into non stick baking tin (approximately 9″ × 6″).
+ Bake at 190°C/375°F/gas mark 5 for 15 minutes.
+ Cut into 8 bars.

Nutritional information (per bar):
Calories = 203; protein = 5.8 g; carbohydrate = 32 g; fat = 6.5 g; fibre = 2.7 g

Muesli Bars

Makes 16 bars

2 oz (50 g) butter or margarine
3 tbsp (45 ml) honey
3 oz (75 g) muesli
3 oz (75 g) wholemeal flour (self
raising)

2 eggs
8 fl oz (225 g) low fat natural
yoghurt
8 oz (225 g) low fat soft cheese
4 oz (100 g) mixed dried fruit

+ Combine butter and honey.
+ Mix in yoghurt, soft cheese and eggs, followed by remaining ingredients.
+ Spoon into non stick baking tin (approximately 12″ × 7″).
+ Bake for 20–25 minutes or until firm and golden.
+ Slice into 16 bars.

Nutritional information (per bar):
Calories = 112; protein = 4.8 g; carbohydrate = 14 g; fat = 4.5 g; fibre = 0.9 g

Real Fruit Cake

Makes 10 large slices

2 apples or pears, grated
1 banana, mashed
4 oz (100 g) sultanas
2 oz (50 g) chopped dates
2 oz (50 g) dried ready-to-eat
   apricots
¼ pint (150 ml) orange juice

3 eggs
1 tbsp (15 ml) honey
4 oz (100 g) wholemeal flour
4 oz (100 g) cornmeal or white
   flour
1 tbsp (15 ml) baking powder
¼ pint (150 ml) skimmed milk

- Mix all ingredients together.
- Spoon mixture into non stick, 8″ round cake tin.
- Bake at 160°C/350°F/gas mark 4 for approximately 1 hour or until firm to the touch.

Nutritional information (per slice):
Calories = 176; protein = 5.6 g; carbohydrate = 34 g; fat = 2.7 g; fibre = 2.3 g

Variations:

Substitute any of the following for the equivalent weight in the recipe: Dried mango slices; dried tropical fruit mixture; tinned pineapple/mango/apricots/cherries; fresh or dried blueberries or cranberries; dried pineapple/papaya pieces; figs; ready-to-eat prunes; plums; fresh, tinned or dried peaches.

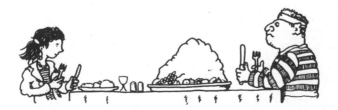

Index

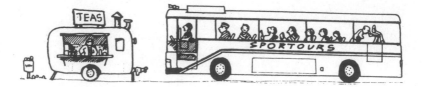

Published by A & C Black (Publishers) Ltd
35 Bedford Row, London WC1R 4JH

Second edition 1996
First edition 1993
Reprinted 1994, 1995

Copyright © 1993, 1996 by Anita Bean

ISBN 0 7136 4388 9

A CIP catalogue record for this book
is available from the British Library.

Acknowledgements
The author would like to thank Simon Bean, Peggy Wellington,
Andy Jackson and Gillian Gale for their invaluable help in this project.
Cover photograph courtesy of Tony Stone Images.

Distributed in the USA by
The Talman Company
131 Spring Street
New York, NY 10012.

Photoset in 11 on 13 pt Palatino by Rowland Phototypesetting Limited,
Bury St Edmunds, Suffolk
Printed and bound in Great Britain by
WBC Book Manufacturers, Bridgend